The NATURAL PHARMACY

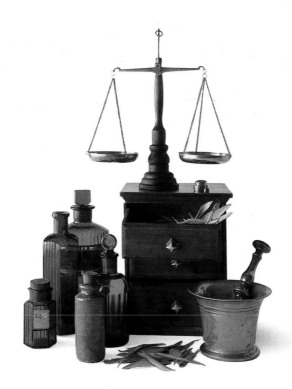

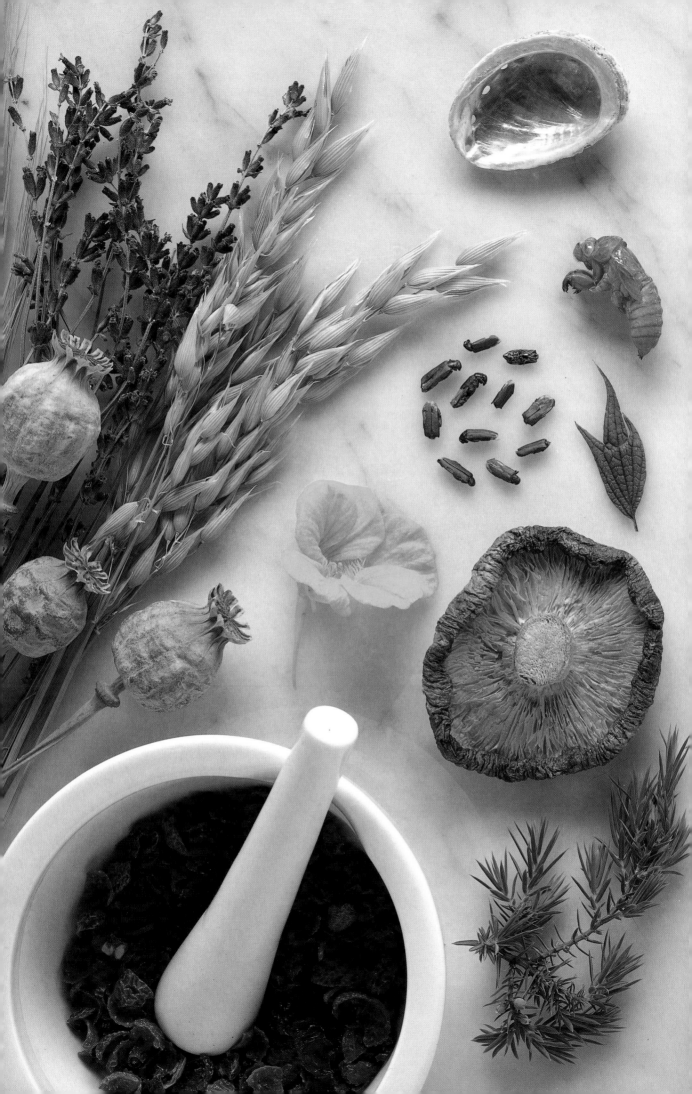

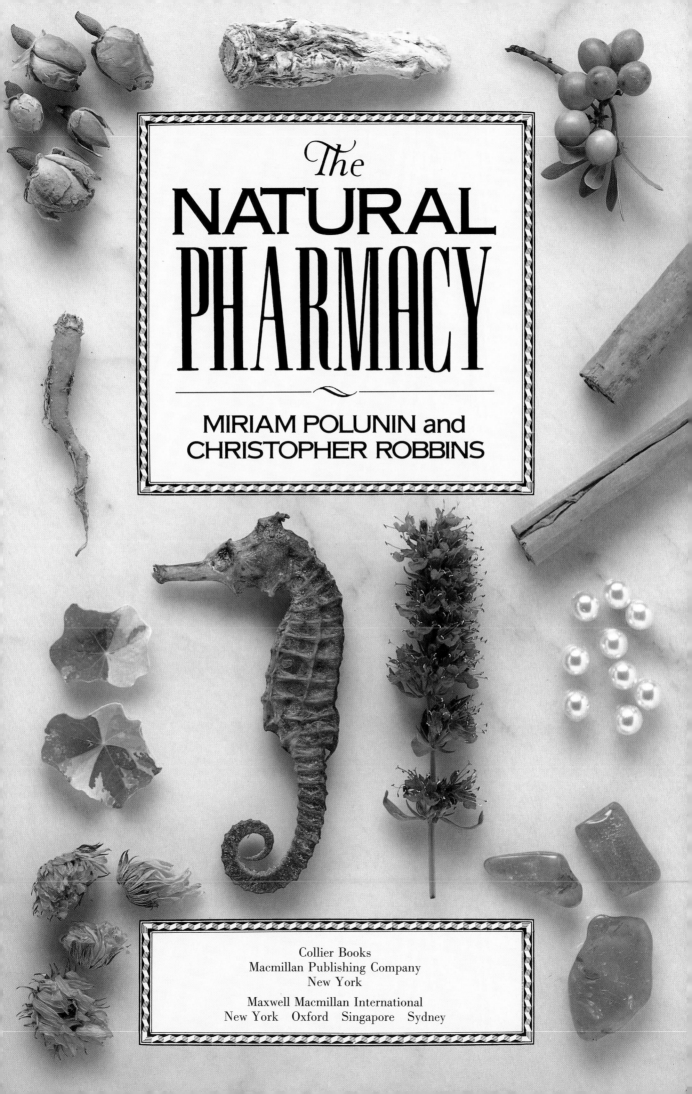

The
NATURAL
PHARMACY

MIRIAM POLUNIN and
CHRISTOPHER ROBBINS

Collier Books
Macmillan Publishing Company
New York

Maxwell Macmillan International
New York Oxford Singapore Sydney

A DORLING KINDERSLEY BOOK

Editor Helen Barnett • **Art Editor** Karen Ward • **Senior Editors** Carolyn Ryden &
Rosie Ford • **Senior Managing Editor** Daphne Razazan • **Managing Art Editor**
Carole Ash • **Production** Antony Heller • **Photography** Steve Gorton

Important Notice

This book is not a medical reference book. The advice it contains is general, not specific
to individuals, and neither the authors nor the publishers can be held responsible for any
adverse reactions to the remedies, recommendations, or instructions contained herein. Do
not try self-diagnosis or attempt self-treatment for serious or long-term problems without
consulting a qualified practitioner. Do not undertake any self-treatment while you are
undergoing a course of medical treatment without first seeking professional advice.

•

Publisher's note. In this book the terms "ingredients" and "substances" are used to describe the
plants, animals, and minerals, or parts thereof, used in medicine.

First published in Great Britain in 1992
by Dorling Kindersley Limited
9 Henrietta Street, London WC2E 8PS

Collier Books
Macmillan Publishing Company
866 Third Avenue
New York, NY 10022

Macmillan Publishing Company is part of the Maxwell Communication Group of Companies.

Library of Congress Cataloging-in-Publication Data
Polunin, Miriam.
    The natural pharmacy/Miriam Polunin and Christopher Robbins.–
1st Collier Books ed.
    p. cm.
    Includes bibliographical references and index.
    ISBN 0-02-036041-X
    1. Naturopathy–Dictionaries. 2. Herbs–Therapeutic use–
Dictionaries. I. Robbins, Christopher. II. Title.
    [DNLM: 1. Medicine. Herbal. 2. Naturopathy. WB 935 P779n]
RZ433.P65 1992
615'.321–dc20
DNLM/DLC
for Library of Congress   91-40545
                                                                      CIP

Macmillan books are available at special discounts for bulk purchases for sales promotions,
premiums, fund-raising, or educational use. For details, contact: Special Sales Director,
Macmillan Publishing Company, 866 Third Avenue, New York, NY 10022

First Collier Books Edition 1992
10 9 8 7 6 5 4 3 2 1
Printed in Germany

Contents

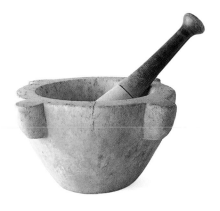

Introduction

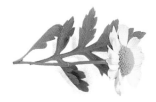

PLANTS, ANIMALS, AND MINERALS have been used to make healing remedies by every human civilization in history. Written records as old as Egyptian hieroglyphics, the Bible, and Chinese herbals detail the extensive use of medicines from nature, and the natural environment remains the major source of healing remedies worldwide. This book explores over 230 of the most significant medicinal plants, animals, and minerals used today.

The World Health Organization has estimated that at least 80 percent of the world's population relies mainly, if not totally, on natural medicines. Even in industrialized countries, up to 40 percent of all pharmaceuticals are derived from natural sources. Many drugs are made with natural ingredients, and others are either synthetic copies or artificially modified forms of natural chemicals.

In industrialized societies, medicines from natural sources are increasing in popularity, not as a "new age" creation but as a re-emergence of an ancient and universal practice from behind the recent shadow of the pharmaceutical industry. There are many reasons for this renaissance. Only in the last 100 years has orthodox medicine come to depend on man-made chemicals that do not occur in nature. Such modern drugs made a dramatic impact on infectious diseases in the 1940s and 1950s, but they have not provided cures for common diseases like breast, lung, or bowel cancers, heart disease, rheumatism, or the common cold. Meanwhile, concern about the frequency and seriousness of drug side effects has grown.

The realization that modern drugs are no panacea, and may cause illness as often as cure it, has coincided with a growth in international awareness of environmental exhaustion and destruction. This has brought greater sensitivity to the intricate webs of interdependence between living things, and a greater appreciation of holistic health philosophies and natural medicines.

Man's knowledge of the healing properties of plants, animals, and minerals is a remarkable testament to the cultural and intellectual evolution of human civilization. The briefest reflection on our ignorance of the world is enough to make us marvel at how primitive societies discovered the healing powers of the things around them. Even more extraordinary is how the same or closely related plants, for example, have been used for the same illnesses by communities thousands of miles apart, when there has been no evidence of communication to transfer knowledge.

Without even a pencil to record their findings, our ancestors must have applied some extraordinary powers of observation and intuition to discover the medicines in nature. The ancients had no laboratories or computers with which to test their remedies, yet they perhaps put them to far more detailed practical evaluation than any modern drug. Every family in every community that used medicines was, in effect, testing them, and only remedies that were considered effective and safe were passed on to the next generation. Over thousands of generations, the therapeutic properties of plants, animals, and minerals were thus subjected to continuous assessment and evaluation. So, it is not surprising that modern science regularly confirms healing actions that were discovered centuries ago.

Healing has usually been intertwined with myth, religion, and power. We may scorn some of the ancient superstitions that surrounded it but, in their time, these provided reasonable explanations for the mysteries of the world, given the limited resources that our ancestors had available to them. Even today, with our greater and more detailed knowledge of the world, superstitions persist and religions still offer spiritual explanations of the mysteries of the world and of life itself.

Although the same remedies may still be used in different parts of the world, they are often used in different ways in different systems of healing. Systems such as traditional Chinese medicine and Ayurveda from India differ from orthodox medicine in being holistic, or treating the whole person. They explain health as being a state of harmony, or balance, both within the body and between each individual and the surrounding environment. Illness is due to imbalance, and remedies are applied to restore harmony.

There are thousands of interesting and important medicines from nature. The plants, animals, and minerals included in this book were selected to emphasize those that either are in current use somewhere in the world or had a dramatic impact on medicine in their day. The choice also reflects the wide range of conditions for which medicines from nature are used. We have excluded remedies which, while still in use, are taken from species facing extinction, for example, musk deer, pangolin, whales, and rhinoceros.

There is irony in the fact that the largest pharmaceutical companies in the world are now sending teams of scientists scrambling through the South American jungles looking for natural sources for future drug products. There are signs that such close contact with the natural harmony of wild places may lead to a greater appreciation of the use of the natural medicines found there. It may increase the understanding of the value of looking at both illness and healing in relation to the whole person and to their interaction with the environment. The natural world will continue to ease the pains and consequences of living in the most modern societies.

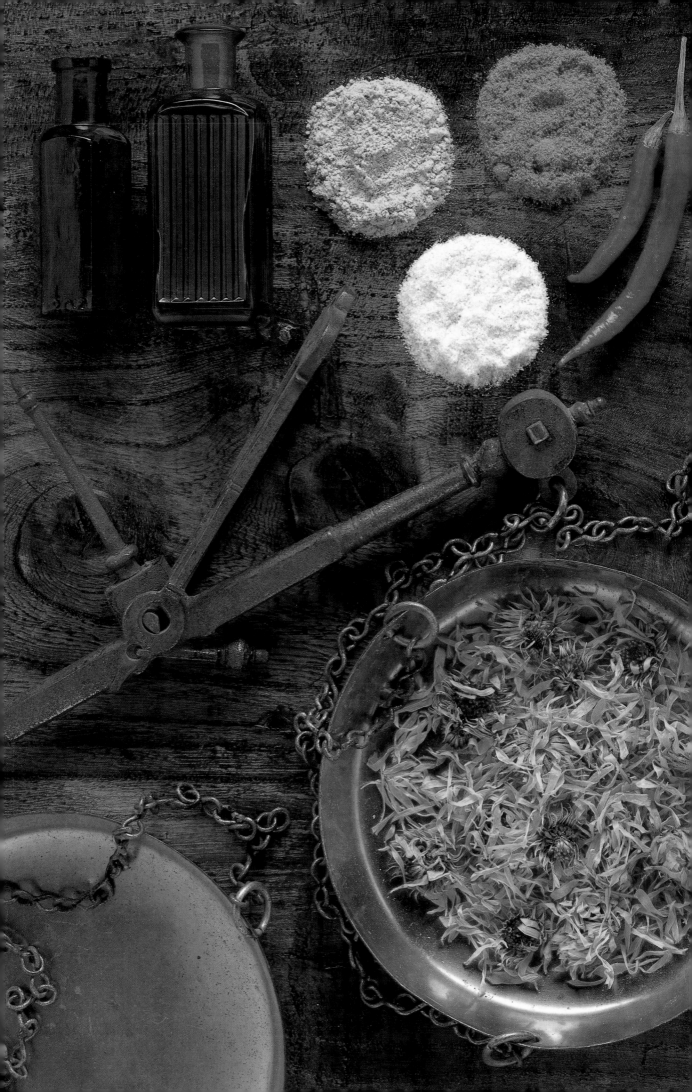

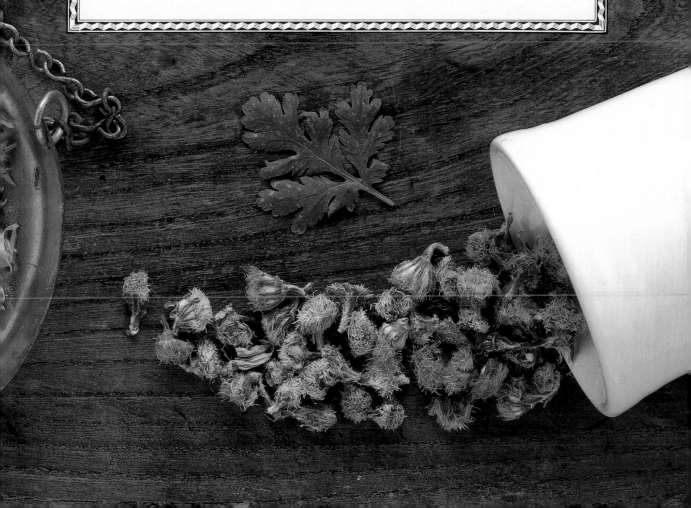

Systems of
Medicine
Past & Present

The spread and development of medicine from
the earliest beginnings, with a guide to the methods and
ingredients used in key systems of medicine.

History of Medicine

A LL HUMAN SETTLEMENTS or civilizations have used the natural environment as a source of healing remedies. The earliest written records of medicine date back about 3,500 years, but paleontologists have found bunches of medicinal herbs among the fossilized remains of our Neanderthal ancestors.

Ancient Civilizations

Surviving Egyptian papyri from around 1,600 BC list a wealth of plant, animal, and mineral remedies, including many still used today. Examples of those listed include plants such as coriander, fennel, gentian, henbane, juniper, pomegranate, senna, thyme, and wormwood; minerals such as aluminum hydroxide, copper, iron, lime, magnesium hydroxide, and mercury; and animal products such as honey, ox liver, wax, and assorted animal fats. At around the same time, clay tablets listing medicinal plants such as castor oil, myrrh, and opium were being produced in Mesopotamia, the fertile triangle between the rivers Tigris and Euphrates. And, in the Chinese Yin dynasty of about 1,500 BC, references to herbal medicine were inscribed on bones (oracle bones), some 160,000 of which have since been uncovered by archaeologists. The Old Testament is also rich in references to medicines from nature, such as mandrake, cinnamon, frankincense, and asafetida.

Egyptian papyrus. Dating from 1,200 BC, this papyrus fragment contains instructions for a headache remedy, including a chant "to be recited over a crocodile of clay with grain in its mouth."

Ancient Egyptian medicine. As far back as 1,600 BC, the Egyptians were recording the use of medicines, as shown here on this stone carving of scribes writing on papyri.

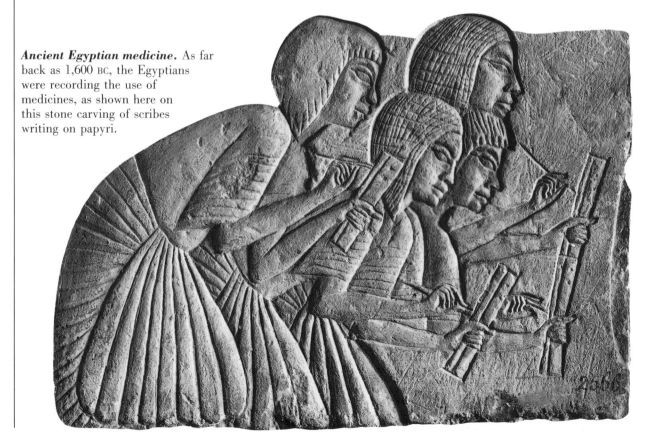

How did early man learn all this? We can only guess that some 300,000 years of interaction with and observation of his environment gradually led to a wide use of plant, mineral, and animal materials to produce certain effects. In all probability, the use of natural remedies began before our ancestors became recognizable as humans. Animals instinctively choose the right combinations and quantities of food they need to stay healthy, know what poisonous plants to avoid, and may know what to consume when ill, and some of this intuitive behavior would have been passed on to early man.

Long before our ancestors could write, certain individuals in any group would have become the most knowledgeable about healing remedies and would have been consulted when it was felt that superior expertise was required. So began the separation of medicine from self-prescribed treatment.

Traditional Chinese Medicine

Veiled in legend, the beginnings of Chinese herbal medicine are reputed to go back more than 5,000 years, but as far as we know, Chinese knowledge of how to use plant, animal, and mineral remedies did not start trickling through to Europe until about the 2nd century AD. However, the use, earlier than this, of many similar remedies in Chinese and Egyptian medicine is striking. Opium and Chinese rhubarb (both traded internationally around the time of Christ), cinnamon, hydnocarpus oil (also used in ancient India), and mercury were common to both.

Even though the remedies used in the East and West still bear similarities, the thinking behind their applications no longer does. Both systems began with the idea that health comes from a balance between the essential elements that make up man's nature, but by the 16th century most European doctors had moved to a disease-based choice of remedies, or a drug for every ill. Chinese medicine has continued, however, to develop its view of ill health as being due to a lack of harmony between a patient, his circumstances in life, and the world around him.

Central to the Chinese medical system is the idea of five elements in nature – wood, fire, earth, metal, and water – that, combined with the theories of Yin and Yang, and of Qi (energy or life force), is used to explain every change and activity in and between man and his environment. The Chinese five elements system parallels systems in Ayurvedic and early Greek medicine which evolved at about the same time.

Other aspects of Chinese medical knowledge were far more advanced than those in the West. Striking examples of Chinese skill include their establishment of the circulation of blood in the body some 2,000 years before the West, and their ability by the 7th century to recognize diabetes and by the 10th century to inoculate against the infectious disease smallpox. In addition, more than 800 years before the West had even invented a printing press, a printed herbal had been distributed throughout China.

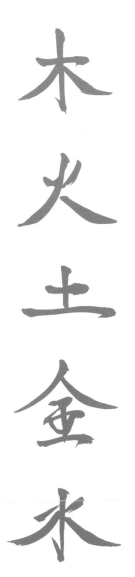

The five elements. These Chinese characters depict wood, fire, earth, metal, and water – the five elements still employed in the diagnosis and treatment of illnesses in traditional Chinese medicine today.

11

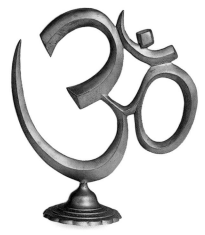

Om. This symbol denotes the life force in Ayurvedic medicine and is often used as a focus in meditation.

Indian herbal. Written in Persian, this medicinal herbal dates back to 17th-century India at the time of the Mogul empire.

The Ayurveda of India

Ayurvedic medicine is another system that is thought to have developed earlier than medicine in the West. Like Chinese medicine, it has kept much the same form throughout its history. It too views health as a balance between a person and the environment, and is a holistic system that takes into account climate, work, eating habits, exercise, emotions, spirituality, and even sexual activities. The theory of the Ayurvedic five elements – earth, air, fire, water, and ether – again suggests communication with other cultures such as ancient Greece. Ayurveda, like Chinese medicine, also recognizes a life force, which is known as *prana*.

Because so many Indians are vegetarian, Ayurvedic medicine has comprised mainly plant remedies. Again, the plants used often overlap with those employed in China and the West. Licorice, ginger, pomegranate, myrrh, basil, garlic, turmeric, aconite, and aloe are among many examples common to both ancient and present day healers.

Ayurvedic medicine was neglected during the Mogul empire (16th–19th century), which brought the Greek-Arab tradition of Unani Tibb treatments to India (see p. 26). But folk use of Ayurvedic medicine continued and, with Indian independence from the British after the Second World War, Ayurvedic tradition was and still is given more professional attention.

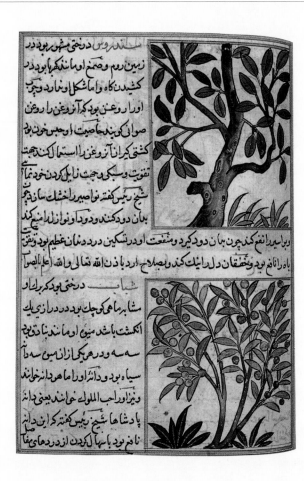

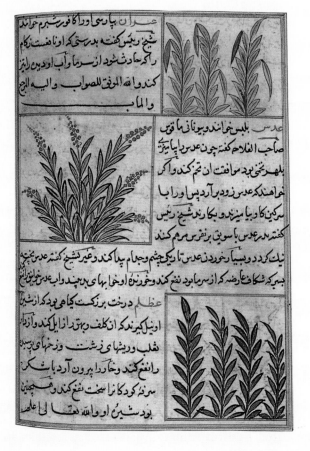

The Growth of Greek Medicine

In ancient Greece in the 5th century BC, Empedocles of Agrigentum began teaching that life rested on four elements – earth, air, fire, and water. It was also held that these corresponded to four humors of the body – black bile, blood, yellow bile, and phlegm. Greek physicians started to work on the principle that good health depended on the right balance of these humors. This theory was the first real concept of a natural rather than supernatural cause of disease and was to dominate medicine in the West for over 2,000 years. Today, we still talk about someone being good or bad humored.

Hippocrates (460–370 BC), who is still referred to as the Father of Medicine, set an excellent example by his methods, which involved studying the patient's individual reaction to a disease and using the patient's own healing powers to correct any imbalance. Treatment was adjusted to the individual and involved diet, massage, water therapy, and rest, as well as plant remedies. Even the best Greek physicians had little knowledge of how remedies worked then, but they watched patients' reactions intently and so built up their skills. By the 3rd century BC, an account of 455 medicinal plants had been produced by Theophrastus. It was probably the first Western herbal, and included many plant remedies still valued today, with details of how to prepare and use them.

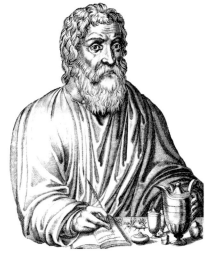

The Father of Medicine.
Hippocrates had a repertoire of some 300 remedies, including many still used today, such as bryony, chamomile, centaury, cassia, garlic, cinnamon, and rosemary. All of these were locally available, and either self-prescribed using local folk knowledge or prepared fresh as recommended by a physician.

Medicine in Roman Times

Roman medicine combined mainly Hippocratic treatments with a heady mixture of magic and religion. But the Romans did make a striking advance in preventive health care by establishing clean water and sewerage by the 6th century BC. They also accepted the idea of infection, isolating infected individuals during epidemics.

Three men seem to have dominated Roman medicine for the first 200 years AD. Celsus wrote a huge guide to medical practice, which included minerals that had been used by the Egyptians, such as mercury, arsenic, and lead. Dioscorides, a Greek in the service of the Roman emperor Nero, produced one of the greatest herbals of all time, with 600 plants described and illustrated in color. Among his descriptions of how to choose and store herbs, he gave a detailed account of how to apply white willow (an early source of aspirin) for pain. Galen, also a Greek working in Rome, was even more influential, but his influence was a mixed blessing. He encouraged Roman officials to check that remedies contained what was claimed, but he also drew up complicated mixtures of herbs known as galenicals. Revived from earlier Egyptian and Greek mixtures, these galenicals were sold at a huge cost as cure-alls and led to fraud for centuries to come. Complicated mixtures with up to a hundred ingredients and generically known as theriacs (from the Greek for antidote) were common during this era.

Roman medicine.
This wooden box dates back to Roman times and was used for carrying medicines, which could be stored individually in the lidded compartments.

13

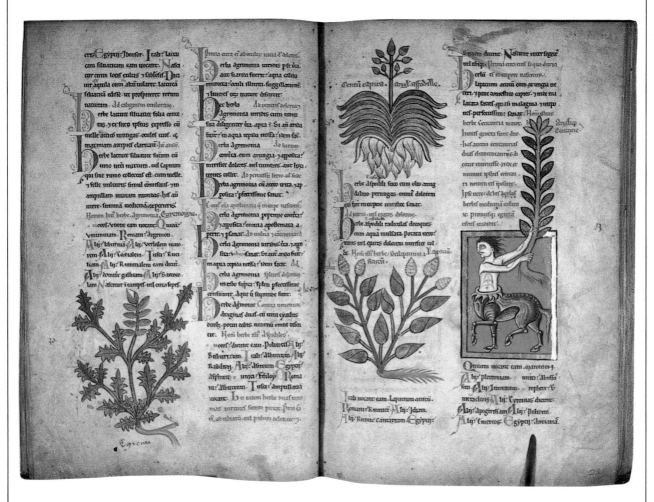

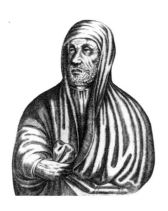

Early herbal. This 12th-century Anglo-Norman manuscript is a fine example of a herbal from Europe's Dark Ages, depicting herbs used medicinally. However, it would have been hard to identify plants safely from such simple images.

Avicenna. Known as the Prince of Physicians, the Persian physician Avicenna wrote a medical text that was to influence medicine the world over for centuries to come.

Islam Takes Up the Torch

Europe's Dark Ages were golden years for Islam. For 1,200 years after the decline of Rome, it was the Muslim empire that kept alive the Greek medical tradition. The Persians and Arabs added remedies such as camphor, musk, nux vomica, and borax, but kept the ideas of Galen. Meanwhile, Judaic views, as might be expected from reading the Old Testament, strengthened the role of public and personal hygiene in the prevention of disease.

The resulting Greco-Islamic medicine was described in an encyclopedia, the *Canon Medicinae*, written in the 11th century by Ibn Sina, the physician now known to us as Avicenna. This knowledge passed west and became the basis for medical treatment at the end of the Dark Ages and for centuries to come. In India, Avicenna's medicine, modelled upon the Greek system of the humors, is still practiced under the name of Unani Tibb; Unani is the Arabic word for "of the Greeks" and Tibb is Arabic for "medicine" and "healing."

In the chaotic Dark Ages of Europe, however, about six centuries passed after the fall of Rome before scientific and medical writing and research revived. During this time, most people had to depend on folk medicine, ritual, and magic in times of ill health. Only the monasteries kept literacy alive, preserving medical and herbal knowledge and laboriously copying manuscripts by hand.

Renaissance – The Birth of New Ideas

The arrival of Byzantine knowledge, the recovery of the European population from the bubonic plague, the voyages of Christopher Columbus, and the invention of printing were among the events that sparked new study in the West of the medical tradition that had been kept alive by Islamic healers. But, while knowledge of the body's structure and workings grew enormously, the ideas of Galen and Avicenna were still so much revered that variations between patients were neglected.

Revolt was led by Aureolius Philippus Theophrastus Bombastus ab Hohenheim (1493–1541), who renamed himself Paracelsus, literally meaning "better than Celsus" (the Roman physician). He built up the Doctrine of Signatures, predicted the discovery of active ingredients in plants, and saw illness as an external event and not an imbalance of humors.

Having worked in mercury mines when a young man, Paracelsus was particularly impressed with metals. He encouraged the use of mercury and antimony treatments, thinking wrongly that he could avoid their harmful effects by refining them. His followers were encouraged by the arrival of drugs from the New World acquired from Native South Americans. Peruvian bark provided quinine, which must have seemed a magical answer to one of the oldest and worst health problems, malaria. And the New World disease of syphilis, which also arrived back with the explorers, seemed a perfect example of an illness needing fierce treatment such as mercury.

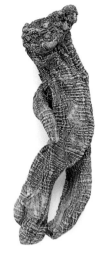

Mandrake. In the Doctrine of Signatures, God was said to provide natural remedies with visible clues for their best use. By resembling the human form, mandrake, for example, was believed to create that form and overcome infertility.

New World medicines. European explorers of the Americas discovered many new sources of medicine, such as ipecacuanha with its dramatic effects on dysentery.

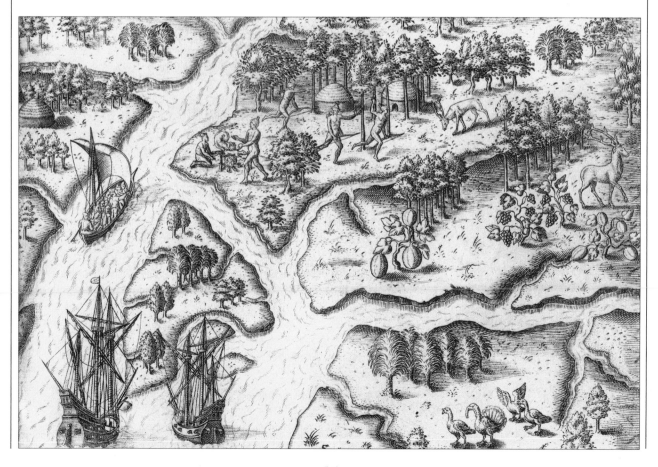

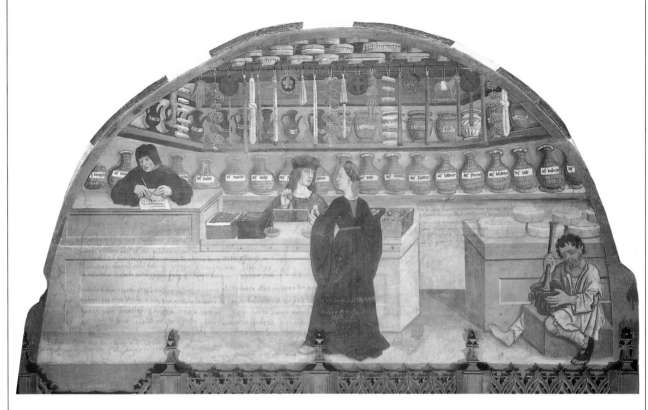

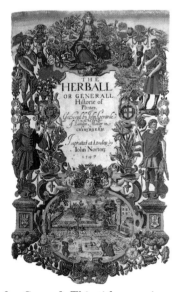

An early pharmacy. This 15th-century fresco, from the Villa Issogna, shows herbalists at work and the types of wares for sale in an early Italian pharmacy.

John Gerard. This title page is from Gerard's famous *The Herball or Generall Historie of Plantes*, which he first published in 1597. The herbal contained descriptions of over 2,000 plants.

Herbals Versus Nightmares

The next 300 years of Western medicine, until the 19th century, sound like a nightmare. While knowledge of the body increased by leaps and bounds, so did populations and cities. Dirty water, contaminated sewers, overcrowding, and grinding poverty combined to give a friendly welcome to all kinds of illness. Drastic treatment, from bleeding to laudanum and mercury to arsenic, was the norm.

Yet the 16th and 17th centuries were also the time when many great herbals were published. The advent of printing made it possible to publish translations of classical Greek and other medical works. And Europe added its own knowledge of plants, including English language classics by William Turner (1568), John Gerard (1597), John Parkinson (1640), and Nicholas Culpeper (1652). During this time, the first studies of the New World were published by Spaniards, while a Portuguese writer wrote an account of Native South American medicine. Although most of the remedies written about were derived from plants, many substances from animals were included, such as snake flesh, earthworms, gallstones from several mammals, and antlers.

Throughout this era, doctors became increasingly able to keep out competing healers. They used their power to enact laws that made practicing medicine a closed shop, and the gulf between doctors and traditional healers widened. But apothecaries, once merely the "grocers" who supplied the medicines prescribed by physicians, gained a growing role. After a 17th-century battle against the physicians' monopoly, they won royal permission to train in medicine and give advice, but were allowed to charge only for the remedies.

Poisons and the Minimum Dose

While mainstream medicine believed many substances to be useful, even if they harmed the patient, some 19th-century doctors were not happy with the drastic doses of substances known to be harmful. The use of mercury was a particular scandal. Given for many illnesses, it even contributed to the deaths of Charles II in 1685 and George Washington in 1799.

In Germany, Samuel Hahnemann (1755–1843), the founder of homeopathy, tried to work out the smallest dose of a remedy that could be given and yet still help the patient. He concentrated on poisonous substances, developing the theory of homeopathy. After years of testing his remedies on himself and friends, Hahnemann started work to establish which doses were most effective. He used smaller and smaller amounts to avoid harmful effects, until he concluded that a single molecule of a substance could be effective, and more so than larger, more damaging amounts.

Native American Medicine

European pioneers venturing to the New World soon sought out indigenous plant remedies, and many of them learned from the Native Americans. Their knowledge of plant remedies was impressive and often included a "like for like" element: the look of the plant was a guide to its application. The use of steam baths and sweating to aid healing and hygiene, and of psychological treatment in the form of ceremonies, was also common. And they were able to teach the settlers about surgical techniques, wound healing, safer methods of birth control, and how to set broken bones. The Native American shamans, or medicine men and women, taught that knowledge of medicine came from dreams, but it was really gathered through careful observation, and trial and error.

While individuals such as John Josselyn, author of the 1672 guide to Native American medicine, *New England's Rarities Discovered*, appreciated this knowledge, orthodox medicine ignored it. Native American plant remedies such as snakeroot, sassafras, dogwood, willow, slippery elm, blue flag, and goldenrod became standard pioneer remedies, but most doctors stuck to the Old World horrors of mercury and bleeding. Washington's death under such treatment coincided with the start of Samuel Thomson's revival of plant medicine in revolt against "heroic" medicine. Although he did not credit them, his techniques of steaming, sweating, and prescribing lobelia and other herbs seemed to be drawn from Native American practices.

But Thomson's methods were also tough on the patient and, by the time homeopathy arrived in the mid-19th century, many Americans were eager to adopt such safe and gentle treatments.

Medicine men. Native American medicine men, who are also shamans, taught that dreams held the secrets of healing. In fact, they had a vast practical knowledge of medicine, which was passed down through the generations.

17

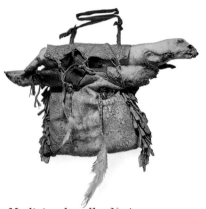

Medicine bundle. Native Americans used bundles like this, which held sacred tobacco, in rituals carried out to boost the fertility and growth of their tribe.

It was a quagmire period of patent medicines, which were based on indigenous American herbs, European purgatives, or both, and on conflicting advice from doctors, travelling medicine men, and folk knowledge. But orthodox medicine soon organized a strong cartel against other methods, and pushed herbalism and homeopathic medicine to a semi-legal fringe.

Today, few of the plants that were learned of from the Native Americans have been adopted by orthodox medicine (although plant-based remedies such as quinine, tubocurarine, aspirin, and reserpine, which originated from other cultures, have been). Meanwhile, herbalists and those who rely on folk knowledge, both in North America and Europe (where Native American remedies had a strong influence in the past), quietly continue using indigenous American herbs for a wide range of healing purposes in their daily practice.

Drugs of the 19th Century

Although the idea of isolating people who were ill had been established since Roman times, it was not until the 19th century that Western medicine fully grasped the link between hygiene and health. Cities began to put in sewers and water systems to match the standards of ancient Rome. Inoculation against smallpox by Jenner tackled an enormous threat, and Pasteur and Koch widened knowledge of how to immunize against other infectious diseases at a time when half of all adult deaths were due to tuberculosis. During the same period, anesthesia was invented, Lister established sterile surgery, and health generally began to improve.

At the turn of the 19th century, natural materials were still universally used and many were at the center of medical advance: for example, cinchona for malaria, foxglove for heart complaints, chloroform from the distillation of alcohol with chlorinated lime for anesthesia, and carbolic acid from coal tar for cleaning. All these remedies have benefited the health of millions since but there were also less helpful natural items such as mercury, which still persisted as treatment for syphilis, or strychnine from the nux vomica plant. As scientific knowledge improved, it was possible to put into action the ambition to extract from plants their active ingredients, something Paracelsus had once dreamed of. The breakthrough in this was the analysis of a particular substance in opium, morphine, in 1803 by a 20-year-old pharmacy apprentice in Germany, Friedrich Serturner. Then, in 1819, atropine was isolated from belladonna, followed by hyoscine, both of which are nerveblockers with many medical uses. In 1820, the antimalarial quinine was isolated from Peruvian bark and, in 1829, emetine from ipecacuanha to provide a valuable emetic. In 1860, cocaine was extracted from coca leaves, providing a local anesthetic that made many operations possible. The next step was to synthesize substances in the laboratory, making either a copy

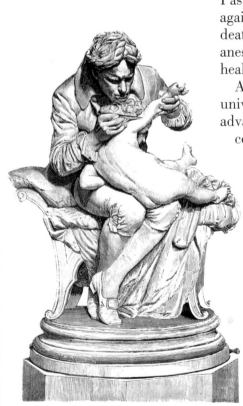

Edward Jenner. A parson's son, he discovered how to vaccinate against smallpox in 1796. This sculpture by Monteverde shows him carrying out his first vaccination.

of the chemical structure of a natural active ingredient or creating a completely new structure not found in nature. A classic example of this was the synthesis of aspirin. In 1827, a French chemist had isolated an active ingredient from meadowsweet that he named salicin, which traditional medicine had been using unknowingly throughout the centuries in willow bark. In 1899, acetylsalicylic acid (aspirin) was derived from salicin, and soon it was being synthesized in the laboratory without the need of meadowsweet.

The 20th Century and Beyond

Within the last 90 years, the use of natural medicines has become the exception rather than the rule in industrial societies, and pharmaceutical drugs have taken over. In the same period, improvements in public hygiene and housing, surgical techniques, immunization, and preventive health care have given orthodox medicine the aura of complete success. But many people find it does not have the answer for them, and basic problems remain: powerful drugs may have serious side effects and still not cure a patient's problem. Should they be seen as superior to traditional remedies? And, should we go on concentrating so much on the treatment of disease rather than strengthening the defenses of an individual against illness? In addition, in most systems of medicine other than orthodox, diet is given equal importance to remedies in treatment. The scientific identification of nutrients in food in the 20th century has helped doctors to identify deficiency problems and plan healthy diets. But it is a relatively new area and much remains to be understood scientifically that traditional healers may know from experience. For instance, in 1897, a Dutch doctor realized that beriberi (inflammation of the nerve endings) was caused by a food deficiency, but the Chinese had recognized beriberi as a deficiency illness and knew what foods patients should eat to correct it as early as the 3rd century AD. As well as nutrients, foods contain many ingredients that have an effect on the body's health-restoring abilities. Such foods include relaxants such as chamomile tea, stimulants such as coffee, tea, and chocolate, digestive stimulants from bitter plants such as chicory, and many more. So what does the future hold? The new awareness of human dependence on the environment may lead to a greater appreciation of the natural medicines found there. In fact, many pharmaceutical companies are already sending teams of scientists to tropical forests around the world in search of new drugs. And more and more people are turning to other systems of medicine, such as homeopathy and herbalism, for relief from their ills.

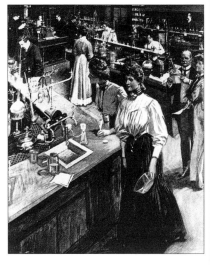

Science develops. A turn-of-the-century laboratory of chemists at work; in the 20th century factory-made drugs rather than natural remedies have become the norm.

Madagascan periwinkle. This rain forest plant has provided two drugs that are effective in the treatment of leukemia and other rare cancers.

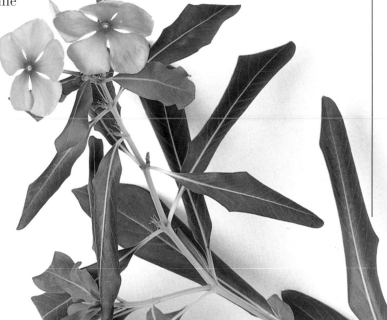

Herbal Medicine

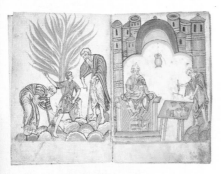

Medieval manuscript of herbalists at work.

MODERN HERBAL MEDICINE combines a holistic philosophy with the exclusive use of plant material. Past medical history and physical, psychological, and environmental factors are assessed for each patient, in order to discover the underlying causes of symptoms. Treatment is not limited to easing symptoms, however, but aims to restore the body's normal functions, so that it can heal itself. For example, treating eczema could involve herbs that act on the liver, kidney, nervous system, and lymphatic system, as well as herbs that soothe the skin and relieve itching. An herbal medicine may comprise a whole plant, parts of a plant (the leaves, stems, flowers, fruit, root, or seeds), or extracts of a plant (such as a tincture or oil). A prescription may consist of a single plant, when it is called a simple, or a mixture of several different herbs. There are over 2,000 medicinal plants to choose from, and, even today, 80 percent of the world's population relies on herbal medicines. Many plant species have had the same uses in different parts of the world since ancient times.

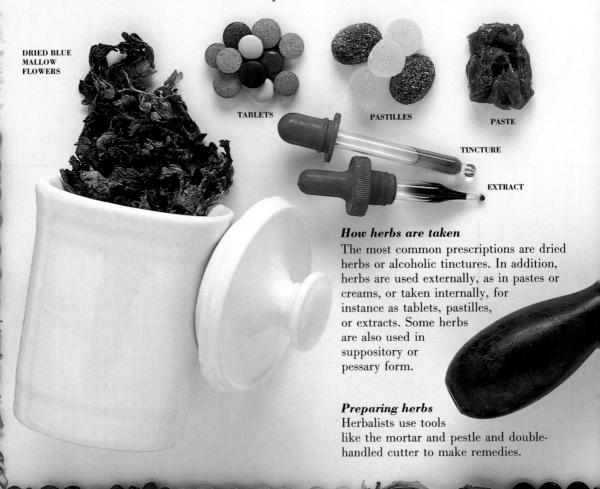

DRIED BLUE MALLOW FLOWERS

TABLETS

PASTILLES

PASTE

TINCTURE

EXTRACT

How herbs are taken

The most common prescriptions are dried herbs or alcoholic tinctures. In addition, herbs are used externally, as in pastes or creams, or taken internally, for instance as tablets, pastilles, or extracts. Some herbs are also used in suppository or pessary form.

Preparing herbs

Herbalists use tools like the mortar and pestle and double-handled cutter to make remedies.

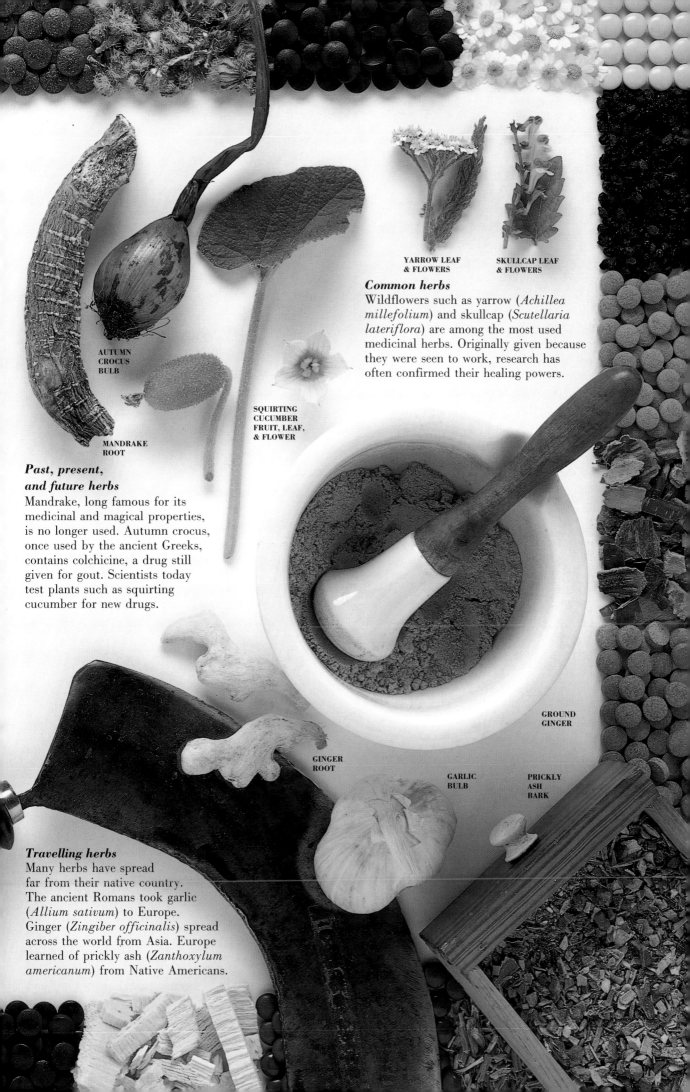

YARROW LEAF & FLOWERS

SKULLCAP LEAF & FLOWERS

AUTUMN CROCUS BULB

MANDRAKE ROOT

SQUIRTING CUCUMBER FRUIT, LEAF, & FLOWER

Common herbs

Wildflowers such as yarrow (*Achillea millefolium*) and skullcap (*Scutellaria lateriflora*) are among the most used medicinal herbs. Originally given because they were seen to work, research has often confirmed their healing powers.

Past, present, and future herbs

Mandrake, long famous for its medicinal and magical properties, is no longer used. Autumn crocus, once used by the ancient Greeks, contains colchicine, a drug still given for gout. Scientists today test plants such as squirting cucumber for new drugs.

GROUND GINGER

GINGER ROOT

GARLIC BULB

PRICKLY ASH BARK

Travelling herbs

Many herbs have spread far from their native country. The ancient Romans took garlic (*Allium sativum*) to Europe. Ginger (*Zingiber officinalis*) spread across the world from Asia. Europe learned of prickly ash (*Zanthoxylum americanum*) from Native Americans.

Chinese Herbalism

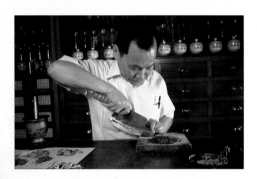

Modern-day Chinese herbalist preparing a remedy.

THE PHILOSOPHY AND PRACTICE of Chinese medicine date back thousands of years, using methods of diagnosis and treatment that are fundamentally different from those in the West. A traditional Chinese physician does not look for a single cause of a disease or symptom but looks for imbalances, or patterns of disharmony, within the whole person. The key to explaining such patterns is known as the Yin-Yang theory, which describes how everything interacts within and with the universe. In addition, the driving force of the body is seen in terms of Qi, or energy, rather than biochemical reactions. Qi exists in different forms, flows throughout the body, and has many functions, such as protecting the body from infection. Types of treatment include acupuncture, herbalism, and moxibustion (heat treatment).

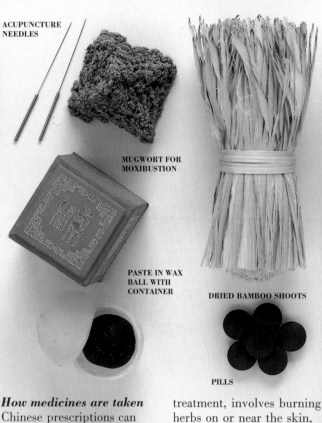

ACUPUNCTURE NEEDLES

MUGWORT FOR MOXIBUSTION

PASTE IN WAX BALL WITH CONTAINER

DRIED BAMBOO SHOOTS

PILLS

GREEN STICKS

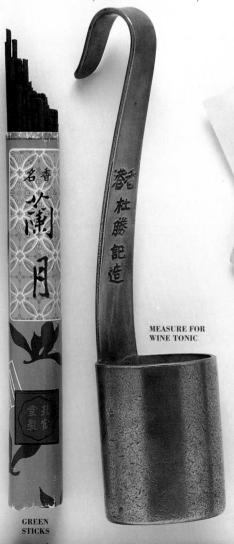

MEASURE FOR WINE TONIC

How medicines are taken
Chinese prescriptions can include up to 20 individual medicines, supplied dried or in the form of broth, tea, powder, pills, or pastes. Tonic wines are served in special measures in herbal stores. Moxibustion, a form of heat treatment, involves burning herbs on or near the skin, or on acupuncture needles; the most used herb for this is Chinese wormwood. Green sticks, which are like incense sticks, are also used to supply heat and to diagnose energy imbalances.

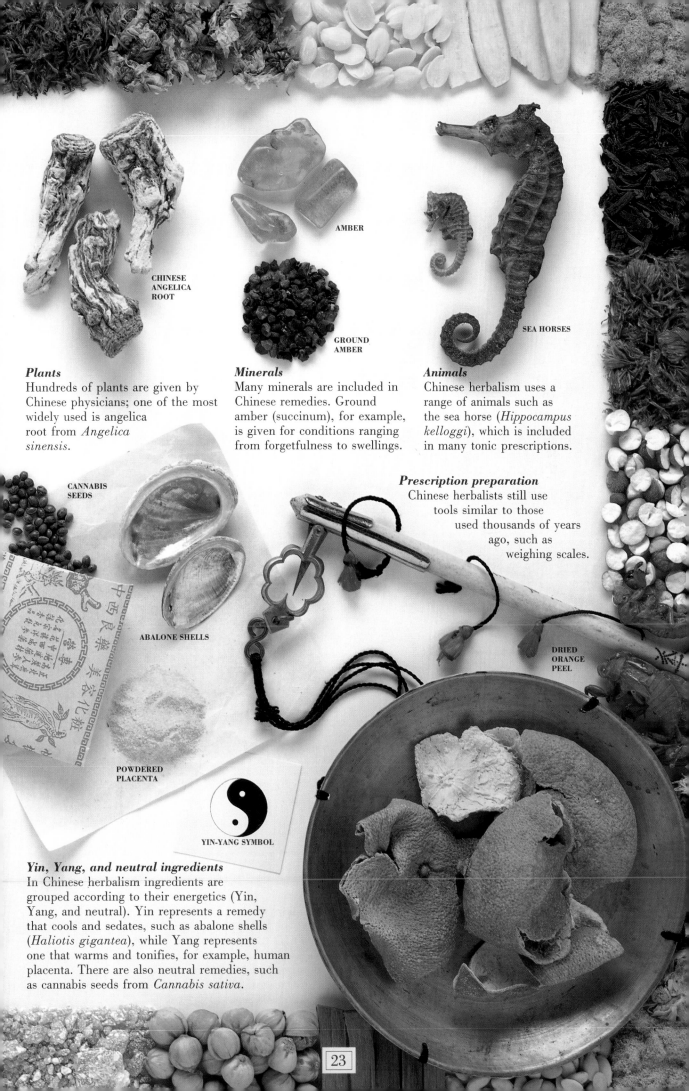

Plants
Hundreds of plants are given by Chinese physicians; one of the most widely used is angelica root from *Angelica sinensis*.

CHINESE ANGELICA ROOT

Minerals
Many minerals are included in Chinese remedies. Ground amber (succinum), for example, is given for conditions ranging from forgetfulness to swellings.

AMBER

GROUND AMBER

Animals
Chinese herbalism uses a range of animals such as the sea horse (*Hippocampus kelloggi*), which is included in many tonic prescriptions.

SEA HORSES

Prescription preparation
Chinese herbalists still use tools similar to those used thousands of years ago, such as weighing scales.

CANNABIS SEEDS

ABALONE SHELLS

POWDERED PLACENTA

YIN-YANG SYMBOL

DRIED ORANGE PEEL

Yin, Yang, and neutral ingredients
In Chinese herbalism ingredients are grouped according to their energetics (Yin, Yang, and neutral). Yin represents a remedy that cools and sedates, such as abalone shells (*Haliotis gigantea*), while Yang represents one that warms and tonifies, for example, human placenta. There are also neutral remedies, such as cannabis seeds from *Cannabis sativa*.

Homeopathy

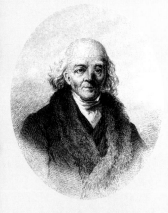

Samuel Hahnemann (1755-1843) – the founder of homeopathy.

A HOMEOPATHIC REMEDY comprises a minute dose of a substance that in large amounts produces the same symptoms from which the patient is suffering. The aim is to stimulate the body's defense mechanisms into fighting the disease. Because such small doses are given – mixtures are diluted until there may be no molecule of the original substance remaining – homeopathy is an unusually safe system of medicine. Many of the 3,000 remedies used are made from plants, minerals, or animals that may be extremely poisonous in large doses. The idea of using "like to treat like" goes back millennia, but it was not until about 200 years ago that the German physician Dr. Samuel Hahnemann founded homeopathic medicine. He experimented to find the smallest dose that would be effective, rather than using the large, often harmful, doses that were popular in orthodox medicine.

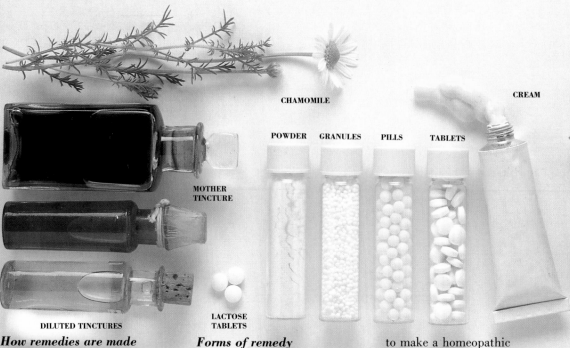

CHAMOMILE

CREAM

POWDER   GRANULES   PILLS   TABLETS

MOTHER TINCTURE

DILUTED TINCTURES

LACTOSE TABLETS

How remedies are made
The ingredient, here chamomile (*Matricaria chamomilla*), stands in alcohol for about a month. One drop of the strained liquid, or mother tincture, is mixed with 99 drops of alcohol and succussed (shaken). Then, one drop of this mixture is added to 99 more of alcohol, and so on. The diluted solution is mixed with lactose.

Forms of remedy
Homeopathic remedies are usually taken in the form of small white tablets or pills which are made of lactose (milk sugar) and have been impregnated with diluted solution. Common dilutions are $6x$ or $30x$. The size of tablet is irrelevant but, surprisingly, the more dilute the solution used to make a homeopathic remedy, the more potent it is. To make a gargle, drops of mother tincture can be used, and people allergic to lactose can buy diluted solutions. Granules or powder is easier for babies to take. Some remedies come as creams or ointments to apply to burns or wounds, for example.

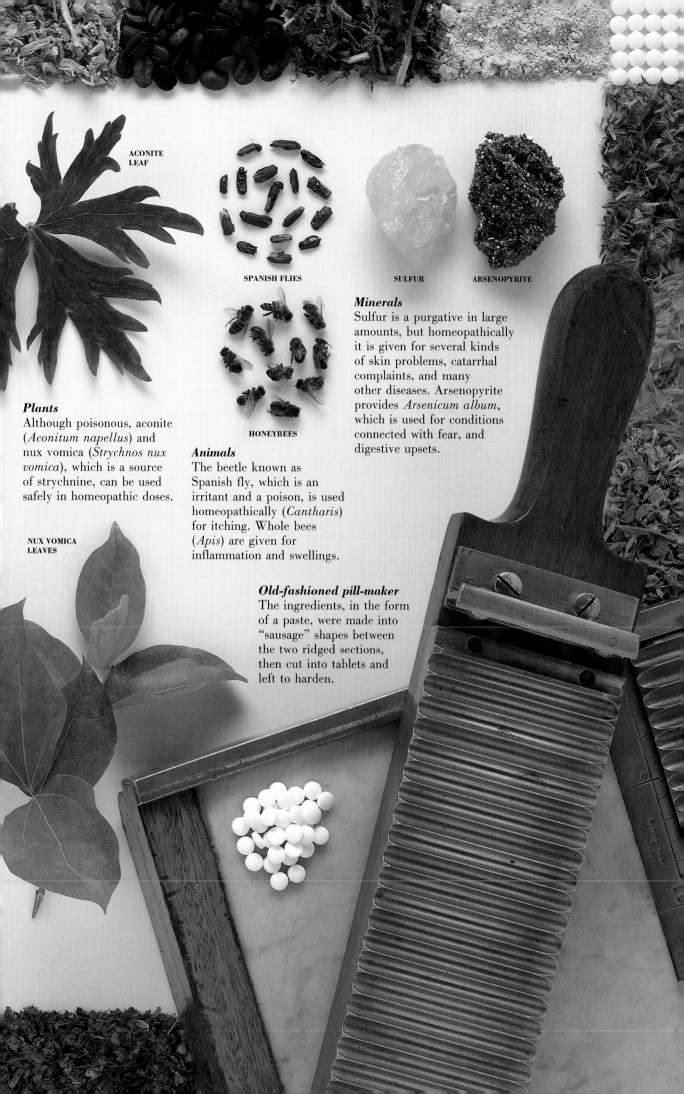

ACONITE LEAF

SPANISH FLIES

SULFUR

ARSENOPYRITE

HONEYBEES

Minerals
Sulfur is a purgative in large amounts, but homeopathically it is given for several kinds of skin problems, catarrhal complaints, and many other diseases. Arsenopyrite provides *Arsenicum album*, which is used for conditions connected with fear, and digestive upsets.

Plants
Although poisonous, aconite (*Aconitum napellus*) and nux vomica (*Strychnos nux vomica*), which is a source of strychnine, can be used safely in homeopathic doses.

Animals
The beetle known as Spanish fly, which is an irritant and a poison, is used homeopathically (*Cantharis*) for itching. Whole bees (*Apis*) are given for inflammation and swellings.

NUX VOMICA LEAVES

Old-fashioned pill-maker
The ingredients, in the form of a paste, were made into "sausage" shapes between the two ridged sections, then cut into tablets and left to harden.

Indian Medicine

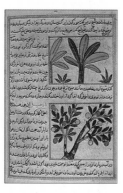

A 17th-century Indian manuscript showing "sour-tasting" fruits.

THE OLDEST SYSTEM of Indian medicine is Ayurveda, meaning "the science of life," which chooses remedies by their ability to harmonize the balance between a patient and the basic influences of life. Ayurveda's view of these influences bears similarities to the other traditional Indian system of medicine, Unani Tibb. Both systems view each individual as being in balance with the influences of earth, air, fire, water, and, for Ayurveda, ether, and both stress preventive health habits. Unani medicine arrived in India with the Mogul empire. It was based on the work of Avicenna (980–1037 AD), the renowned Persian physician who wrote, "Most illnesses arise solely from long-continued errors of diet and regimen." Ayurvedic remedies mainly comprise plants, but also include dairy products, honey, and minerals given in very weak doses, while Unani medicine uses many more animal ingredients.

Ayurvedic Medicine

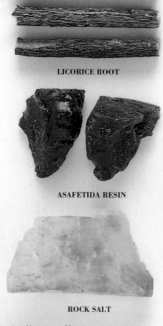

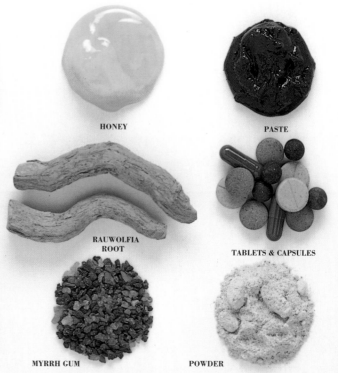

LICORICE ROOT

HONEY

PASTE

ASAFETIDA RESIN

RAUWOLFIA ROOT

TABLETS & CAPSULES

ROCK SALT

MYRRH GUM

POWDER

The six "tastes"
Ayurveda classifies herbs as having one or more of six "tastes," which describe their healing properties. Licorice root from *Glycyrrhiza glabra* is "sweet" and "bitter." Asafetida resin from *Ferula assa-foetida* is "pungent." Rock salt (halite) is "salty." Honey is "astringent" as well as "sweet." Rauwolfia root from *Rauwolfia serpentina* is "bitter." Myrrh gum from *Commiphora molmol* is "bitter" and "pungent." The sixth taste, "sour," comes from fruit.

How remedies are taken
Remedies in Ayurvedic medicine are given either as a paste massaged into the skin, or applied as a poultice, taken in tablet or capsule form, or powdered for use in washes or enemas.

Unani Tibb Medicine

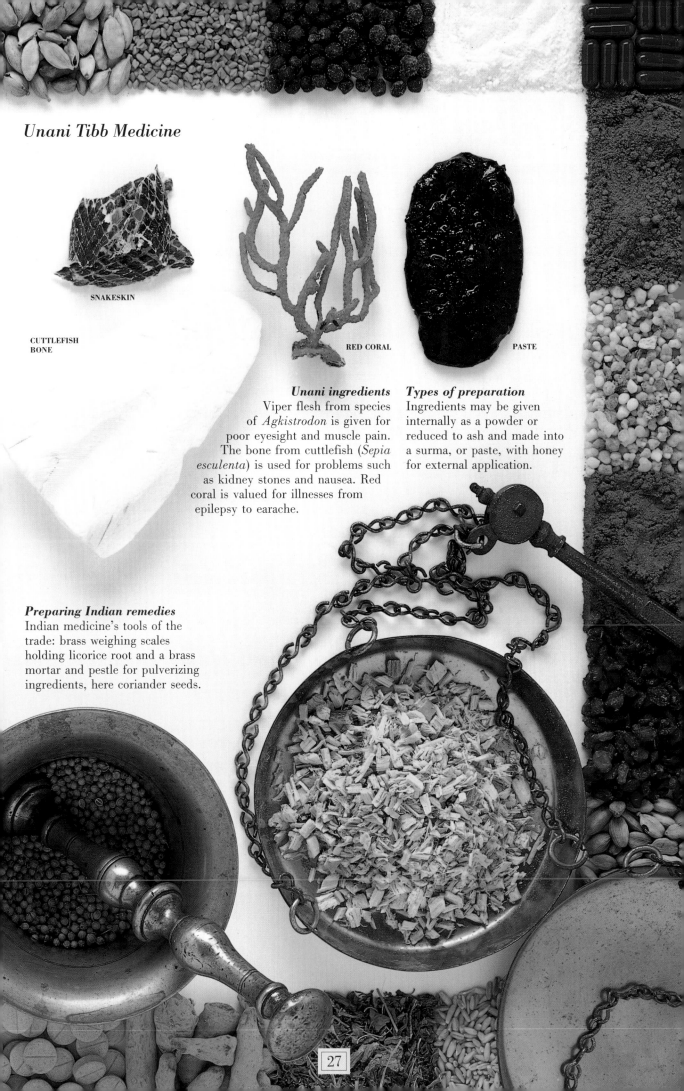

SNAKESKIN

CUTTLEFISH BONE

RED CORAL

PASTE

Unani ingredients
Viper flesh from species of *Agkistrodon* is given for poor eyesight and muscle pain. The bone from cuttlefish (*Sepia esculenta*) is used for problems such as kidney stones and nausea. Red coral is valued for illnesses from epilepsy to earache.

Types of preparation
Ingredients may be given internally as a powder or reduced to ash and made into a surma, or paste, with honey for external application.

Preparing Indian remedies
Indian medicine's tools of the trade: brass weighing scales holding licorice root and a brass mortar and pestle for pulverizing ingredients, here coriander seeds.

Orthodox Medicine

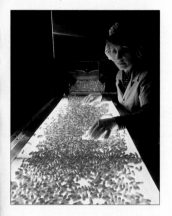

Factory production of drug capsules.

THE DRUGS PRESCRIBED in orthodox medicine contain active substances in precisely measured doses, and are given for a specific symptom or disease. Although man has repeatedly tried to evaluate the medicinally active part of a plant, animal, or mineral, extracting single substances from natural materials was possible only as knowledge of chemistry progressed. Two landmarks in this progress were the extraction of essential plant oils by steam distillation in the 16th century and isolation of the first alkaloid, morphine, from opium poppies in 1803. Now scientists analyze, extract, and copy substances found in nature to produce medicines that are more powerful, safer, cheaper, or easier to provide in a standard dose than their natural sources. Many natural ingredients are still used to make drugs prescribed in orthodox medicine, and many more are being studied as possible sources of drugs.

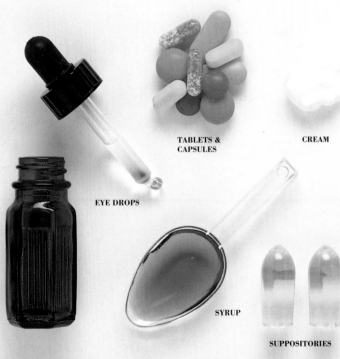

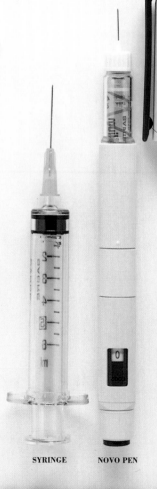

EYE DROPS

TABLETS & CAPSULES

CREAM

SYRUP

SUPPOSITORIES

SYRINGE

NOVO PEN

How drugs are taken

From eye drops and syrups to injections and creams, the ways of giving drugs for the most effective results have been studied almost as widely as the drugs themselves. Suppositories, for example, deliver a drug via the bowel wall that might damage or be rendered ineffective in the stomach. Many natural ingredients provide the carriers for drugs: wax, clays, milk powder, and lanolin. New methods of administering drugs are constantly being developed. The Novo pen, for example, delivers tiny doses of insulin to diabetics before each meal.

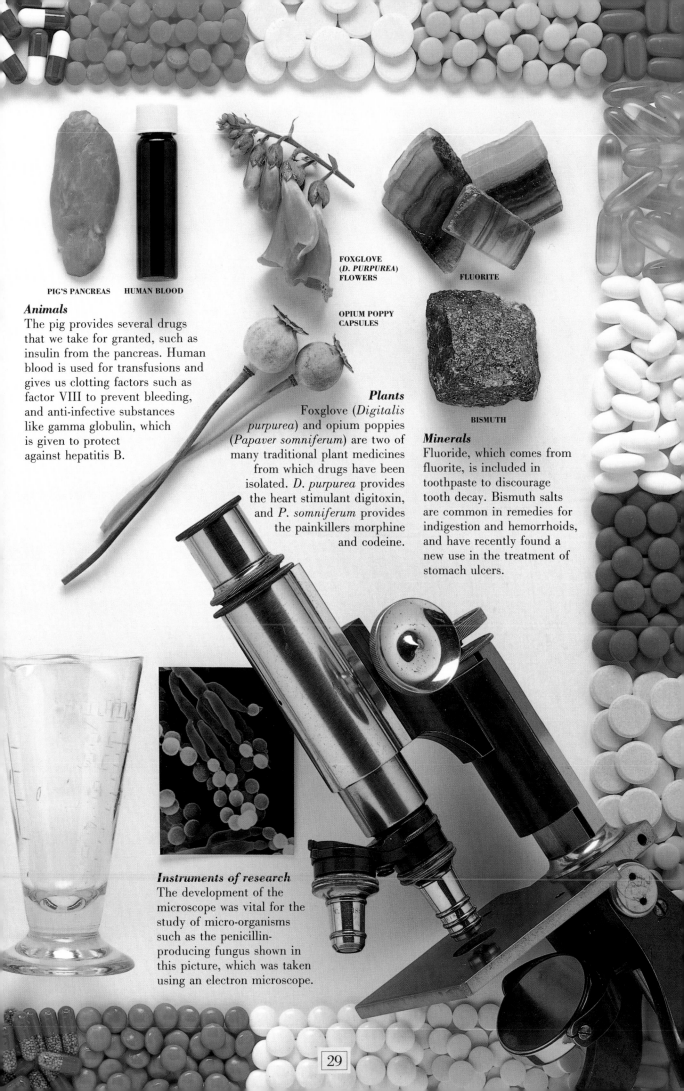

**FOXGLOVE
(*D. PURPUREA*)
FLOWERS**

FLUORITE

PIG'S PANCREAS   **HUMAN BLOOD**

**OPIUM POPPY
CAPSULES**

Animals
The pig provides several drugs that we take for granted, such as insulin from the pancreas. Human blood is used for transfusions and gives us clotting factors such as factor VIII to prevent bleeding, and anti-infective substances like gamma globulin, which is given to protect against hepatitis B.

BISMUTH

Plants
Foxglove (*Digitalis purpurea*) and opium poppies (*Papaver somniferum*) are two of many traditional plant medicines from which drugs have been isolated. *D. purpurea* provides the heart stimulant digitoxin, and *P. somniferum* provides the painkillers morphine and codeine.

Minerals
Fluoride, which comes from fluorite, is included in toothpaste to discourage tooth decay. Bismuth salts are common in remedies for indigestion and hemorrhoids, and have recently found a new use in the treatment of stomach ulcers.

Instruments of research
The development of the microscope was vital for the study of micro-organisms such as the penicillin-producing fungus shown in this picture, which was taken using an electron microscope.

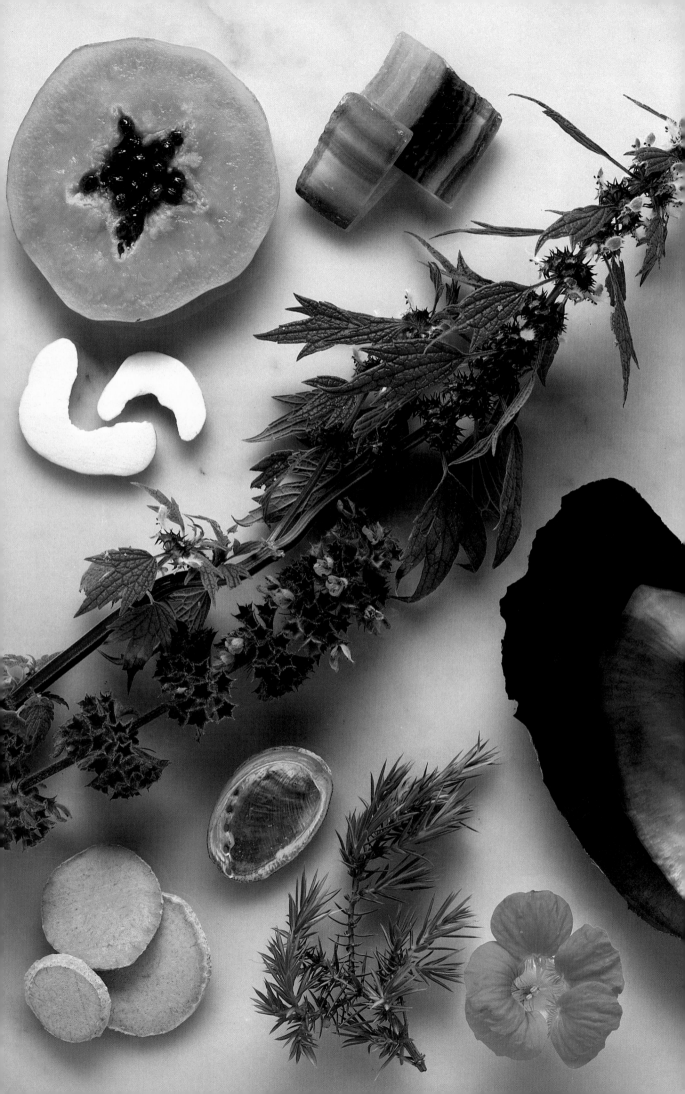

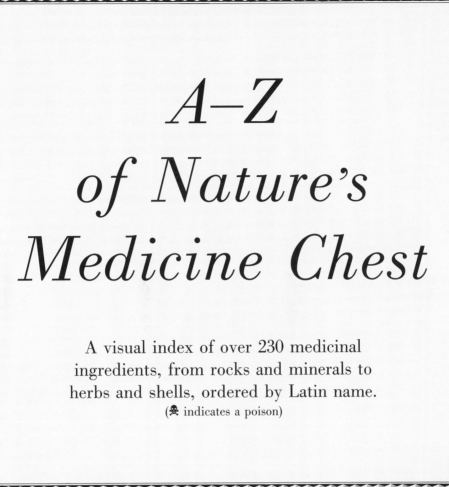

A–Z
of Nature's
Medicine Chest

A visual index of over 230 medicinal
ingredients, from rocks and minerals to
herbs and shells, ordered by Latin name.
(☠ indicates a poison)

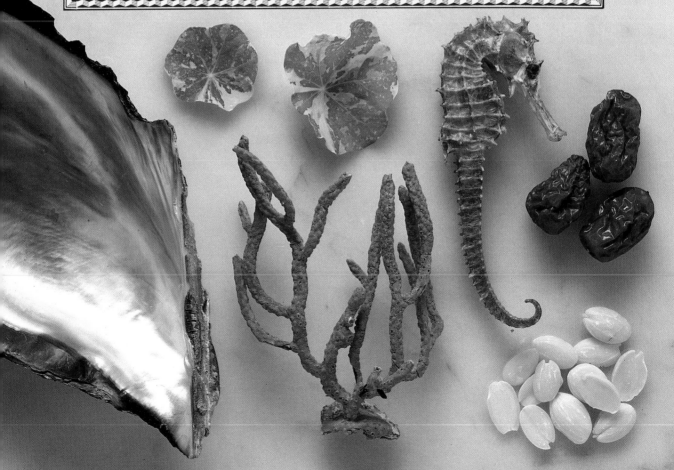

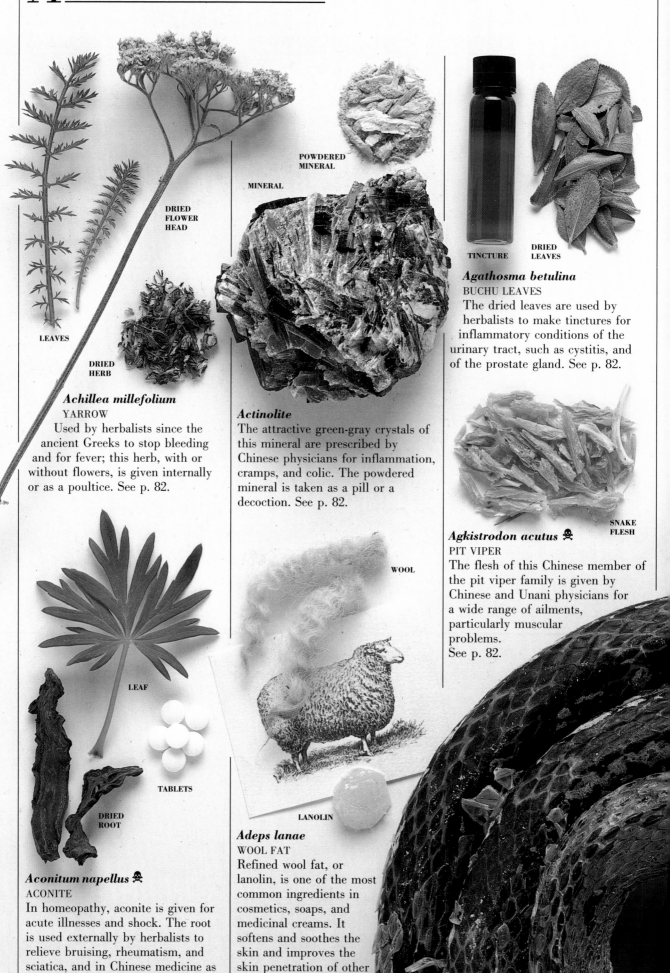

POWDERED
MINERAL

MINERAL

DRIED
FLOWER
HEAD

TINCTURE DRIED
LEAVES

LEAVES

DRIED
HERB

Agathosma betulina
BUCHU LEAVES
The dried leaves are used by
herbalists to make tinctures for
inflammatory conditions of the
urinary tract, such as cystitis, and
of the prostate gland. See p. 82.

Achillea millefolium
YARROW
Used by herbalists since the
ancient Greeks to stop bleeding
and for fever; this herb, with or
without flowers, is given internally
or as a poultice. See p. 82.

Actinolite
The attractive green-gray crystals of
this mineral are prescribed by
Chinese physicians for inflammation,
cramps, and colic. The powdered
mineral is taken as a pill or a
decoction. See p. 82.

SNAKE
FLESH

Agkistrodon acutus ☠
PIT VIPER
The flesh of this Chinese member of
the pit viper family is given by
Chinese and Unani physicians for
a wide range of ailments,
particularly muscular
problems.
See p. 82.

WOOL

LEAF

TABLETS

DRIED
ROOT

LANOLIN

Aconitum napellus ☠
ACONITE
In homeopathy, aconite is given for
acute illnesses and shock. The root
is used externally by herbalists to
relieve bruising, rheumatism, and
sciatica, and in Chinese medicine as
a local anesthetic. See p. 82.

Adeps lanae
WOOL FAT
Refined wool fat, or
lanolin, is one of the most
common ingredients in
cosmetics, soaps, and
medicinal creams. It
softens and soothes the
skin and improves the
skin penetration of other
ingredients. See p. 82.

ALLIUM SATIVUM

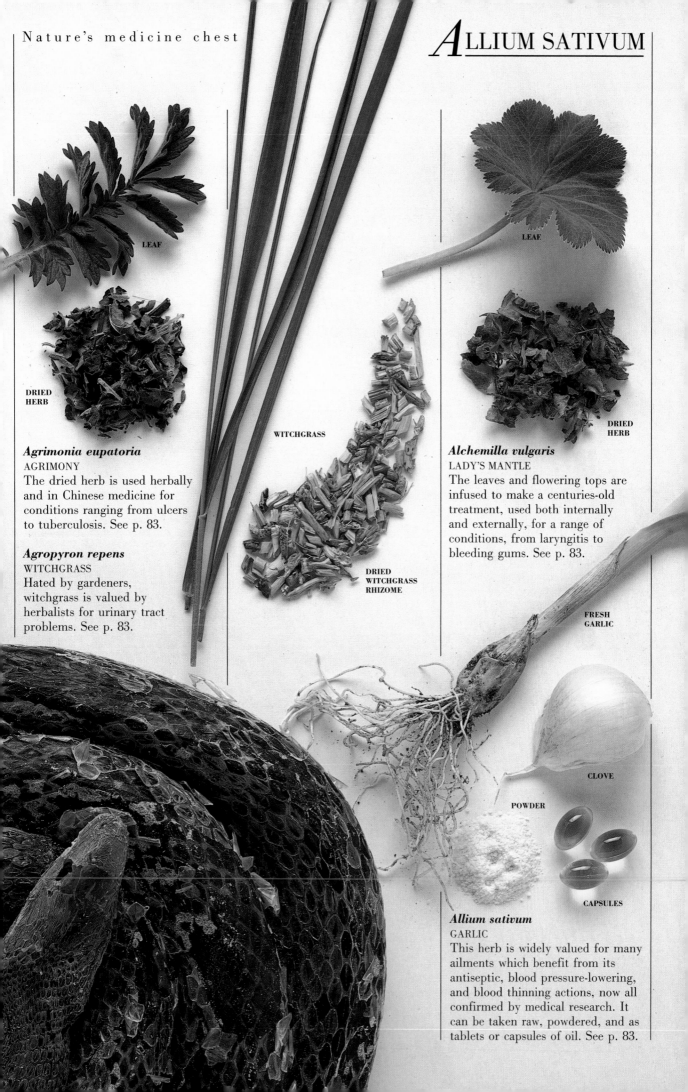

LEAF

DRIED
HERB

WITCHGRASS

DRIED
WITCHGRASS
RHIZOME

LEAF

DRIED
HERB

FRESH
GARLIC

CLOVE

POWDER

CAPSULES

Agrimonia eupatoria
AGRIMONY
The dried herb is used herbally
and in Chinese medicine for
conditions ranging from ulcers
to tuberculosis. See p. 83.

Agropyron repens
WITCHGRASS
Hated by gardeners,
witchgrass is valued by
herbalists for urinary tract
problems. See p. 83.

Alchemilla vulgaris
LADY'S MANTLE
The leaves and flowering tops are
infused to make a centuries-old
treatment, used both internally
and externally, for a range of
conditions, from laryngitis to
bleeding gums. See p. 83.

Allium sativum
GARLIC
This herb is widely valued for many
ailments which benefit from its
antiseptic, blood pressure-lowering,
and blood thinning actions, now all
confirmed by medical research. It
can be taken raw, powdered, and as
tablets or capsules of oil. See p. 83.

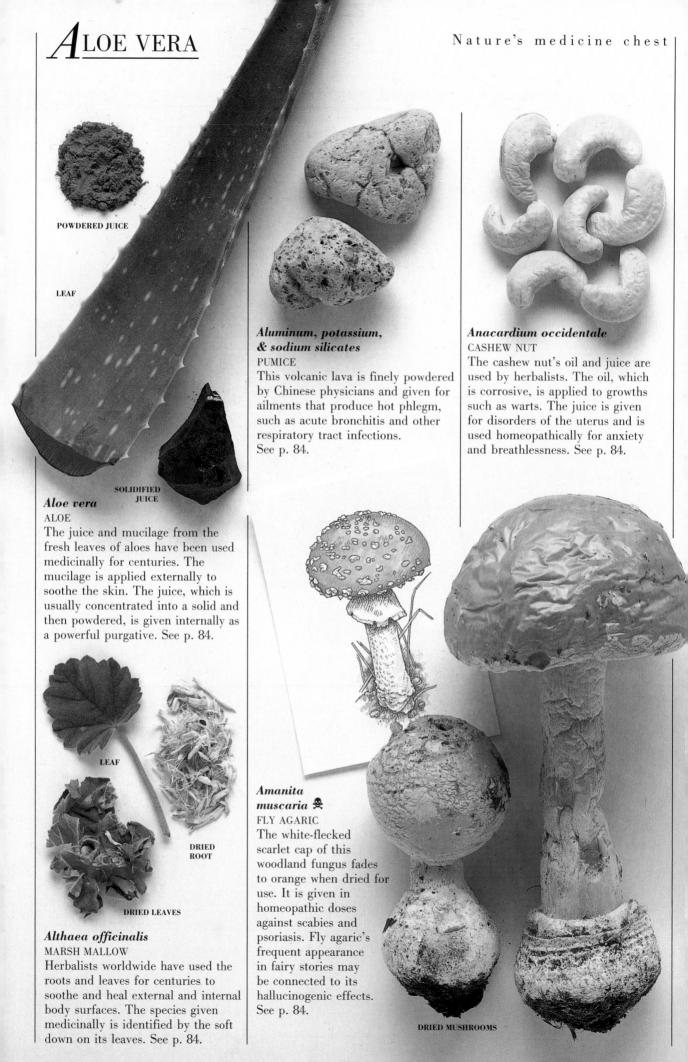

POWDERED JUICE

LEAF

Aluminum, potassium, & sodium silicates
PUMICE
This volcanic lava is finely powdered by Chinese physicians and given for ailments that produce hot phlegm, such as acute bronchitis and other respiratory tract infections.
See p. 84.

Anacardium occidentale
CASHEW NUT
The cashew nut's oil and juice are used by herbalists. The oil, which is corrosive, is applied to growths such as warts. The juice is given for disorders of the uterus and is used homeopathically for anxiety and breathlessness. See p. 84.

SOLIDIFIED JUICE

Aloe vera
ALOE
The juice and mucilage from the fresh leaves of aloes have been used medicinally for centuries. The mucilage is applied externally to soothe the skin. The juice, which is usually concentrated into a solid and then powdered, is given internally as a powerful purgative. See p. 84.

LEAF

DRIED ROOT

DRIED LEAVES

Amanita muscaria ☠
FLY AGARIC
The white-flecked scarlet cap of this woodland fungus fades to orange when dried for use. It is given in homeopathic doses against scabies and psoriasis. Fly agaric's frequent appearance in fairy stories may be connected to its hallucinogenic effects. See p. 84.

DRIED MUSHROOMS

Althaea officinalis
MARSH MALLOW
Herbalists worldwide have used the roots and leaves for centuries to soothe and heal external and internal body surfaces. The species given medicinally is identified by the soft down on its leaves. See p. 84.

APIS MELLIFERA

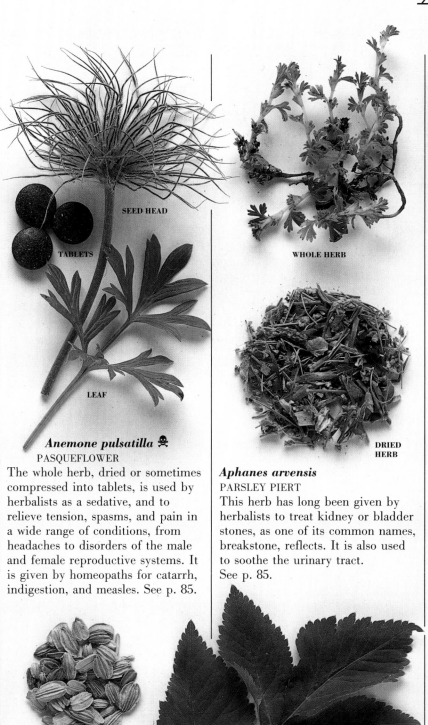

SEED HEAD

TABLETS

LEAF

WHOLE HERB

ROYAL JELLY

BEESWAX

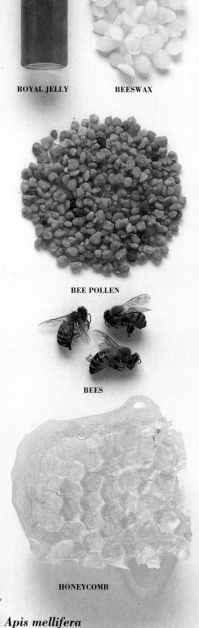

DRIED
HERB

BEE POLLEN

BEES

HONEYCOMB

Anemone pulsatilla ☠
PASQUEFLOWER
The whole herb, dried or sometimes compressed into tablets, is used by herbalists as a sedative, and to relieve tension, spasms, and pain in a wide range of conditions, from headaches to disorders of the male and female reproductive systems. It is given by homeopaths for catarrh, indigestion, and measles. See p. 85.

Aphanes arvensis
PARSLEY PIERT
This herb has long been given by herbalists to treat kidney or bladder stones, as one of its common names, breakstone, reflects. It is also used to soothe the urinary tract.
See p. 85.

DRIED SEEDS

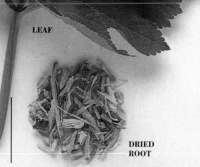

LEAF

DRIED
ROOT

Angelica archangelica
ANGELICA
The dried roots and seeds and fresh leaves and stems of this European variety are used by herbalists – and related varieties by Eastern physicians – for a range of conditions, from flu to indigestion. The name comes from its repute as a treatment for pestilence. See p. 85.

Apis mellifera
HONEYBEE
In Unani medicine, whole bee is given as a tonic and applied to stings. It is given homeopathically for similar complaints. Honey is applied to wounds and burns, and taken for lung complaints and constipation. Beeswax is used like honey in Eastern medicine, and in the West is common in skin creams. Royal jelly is popular as a general tonic. Pollen is taken to build up resistance to hay fever. See p. 85.

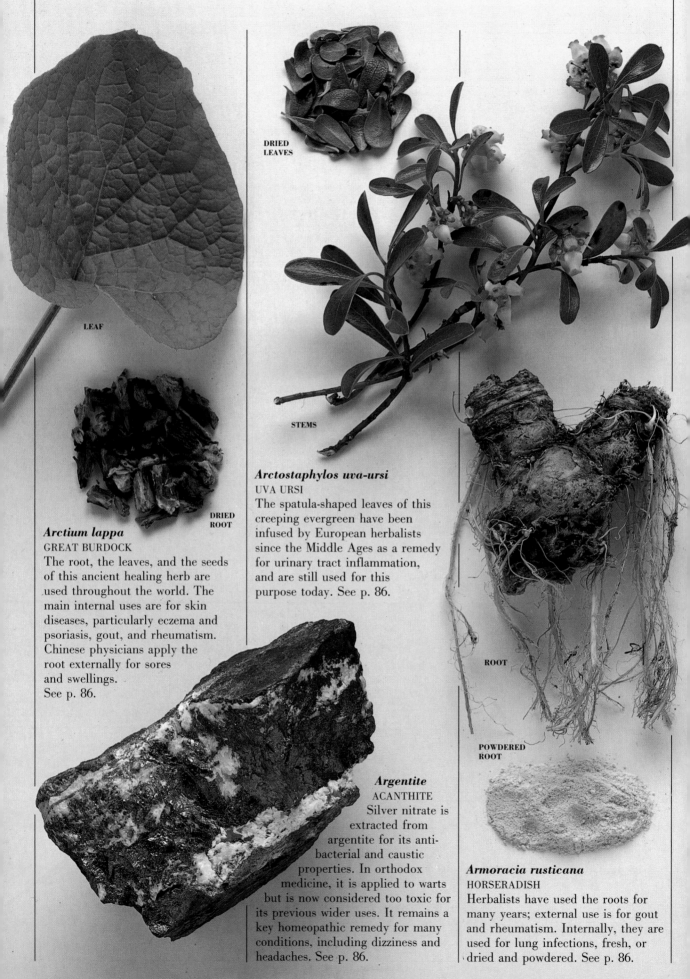

LEAF

DRIED LEAVES

STEMS

DRIED ROOT

ROOT

POWDERED ROOT

Arctium lappa
GREAT BURDOCK
The root, the leaves, and the seeds of this ancient healing herb are used throughout the world. The main internal uses are for skin diseases, particularly eczema and psoriasis, gout, and rheumatism. Chinese physicians apply the root externally for sores and swellings.
See p. 86.

Arctostaphylos uva-ursi
UVA URSI
The spatula-shaped leaves of this creeping evergreen have been infused by European herbalists since the Middle Ages as a remedy for urinary tract inflammation, and are still used for this purpose today. See p. 86.

Argentite
ACANTHITE
Silver nitrate is extracted from argentite for its anti-bacterial and caustic properties. In orthodox medicine, it is applied to warts but is now considered too toxic for its previous wider uses. It remains a key homeopathic remedy for many conditions, including dizziness and headaches. See p. 86.

Armoracia rusticana
HORSERADISH
Herbalists have used the roots for many years; external use is for gout and rheumatism. Internally, are used for lung infections, fresh, or dried and powdered. See p. 86.

*A*SCLEPIAS TUBEROSA

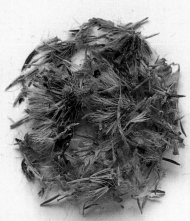

DRIED FLOWER HEADS

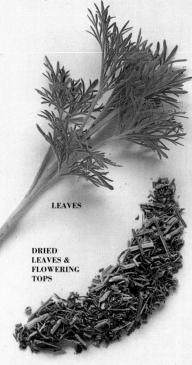

LEAVES

DRIED LEAVES & FLOWERING TOPS

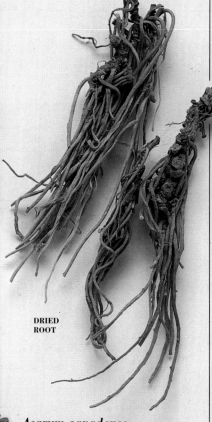

DRIED ROOT

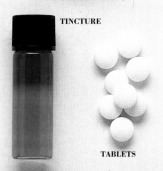

TINCTURE

TABLETS

Arnica montana
LEOPARD'S BANE
This mountain plant is widely taken in homeopathic doses for bruising, wounds, and shock. However, as it is an irritant if taken internally in large amounts, herbalists only apply it externally. See p. 87.

Artemisia abrotanum
SOUTHERNWOOD
The pungent smell of this herb is a key to its use as a bitter. The tops and leaves are used by herbalists for digestive problems. See p. 87.

Asarum canadense
WILD GINGER
The dried root is given by herbalists for flatulent indigestion. Chinese doctors prescribe wild ginger for headaches, toothaches, colds, and bad breath. See p. 87.

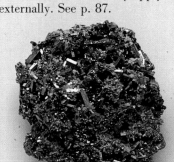

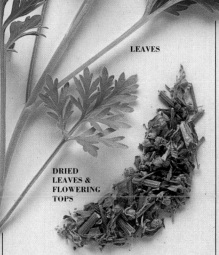

LEAVES

DRIED LEAVES & FLOWERING TOPS

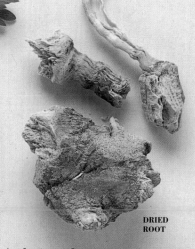

DRIED ROOT

Arsenopyrite ☠
IRON ARSENIC SULFITE
These lustrous metallic crystals are the most important source of arsenic. Homeopaths prescribe *Arsenicum* for food poisoning, psoriasis, thrush, catarrh, and hay fever. Chinese physicians give arsenopyrite for skin diseases, anemia, and asthma. A curious feature of the crystals is that, when struck, they give off a strong smell of garlic. See p. 87.

Artemisia absinthium
WORMWOOD
The leaves and flowering tops are given by herbalists to stimulate the appetite and to eradicate worms. Wormwood has also been used as an insecticide and antiseptic. See p. 87.

Asclepias tuberosa
PLEURISY ROOT
Named after the Greek god of medicine, Asklepios, dried pleurisy root is given by herbalists for ailments such as bronchitis, pleurisy, and flu. Native Americans used it as a food and in ceremonies, as well as a medicine. See p. 88.

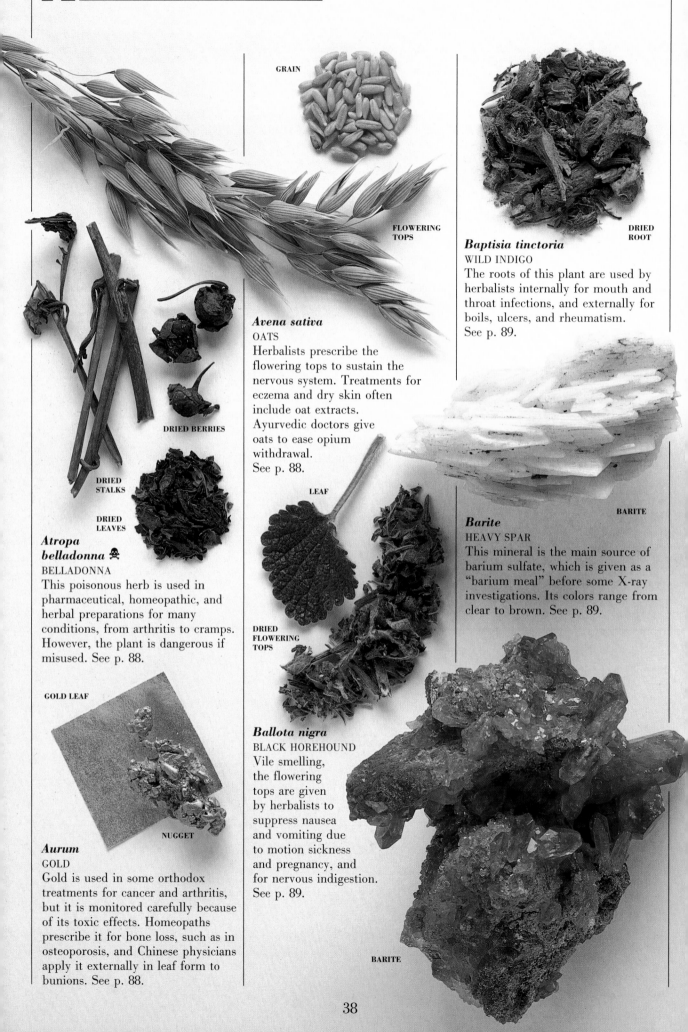

GRAIN

FLOWERING TOPS

DRIED ROOT

Baptisia tinctoria
WILD INDIGO
The roots of this plant are used by herbalists internally for mouth and throat infections, and externally for boils, ulcers, and rheumatism. See p. 89.

Avena sativa
OATS
Herbalists prescribe the flowering tops to sustain the nervous system. Treatments for eczema and dry skin often include oat extracts. Ayurvedic doctors give oats to ease opium withdrawal. See p. 88.

DRIED BERRIES

DRIED STALKS

DRIED LEAVES

LEAF

BARITE

Barite
HEAVY SPAR
This mineral is the main source of barium sulfate, which is given as a "barium meal" before some X-ray investigations. Its colors range from clear to brown. See p. 89.

Atropa belladonna ☠
BELLADONNA
This poisonous herb is used in pharmaceutical, homeopathic, and herbal preparations for many conditions, from arthritis to cramps. However, the plant is dangerous if misused. See p. 88.

DRIED FLOWERING TOPS

GOLD LEAF

Ballota nigra
BLACK HOREHOUND
Vile smelling, the flowering tops are given by herbalists to suppress nausea and vomiting due to motion sickness and pregnancy, and for nervous indigestion. See p. 89.

NUGGET

Aurum
GOLD
Gold is used in some orthodox treatments for cancer and arthritis, but it is monitored carefully because of its toxic effects. Homeopaths prescribe it for bone loss, such as in osteoporosis, and Chinese physicians apply it externally in leaf form to bunions. See p. 88.

BARITE

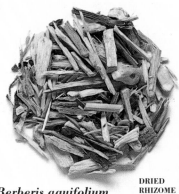

Berberis aquifolium
OREGON GRAPE
The root and rhizome of this shrub, which is a common garden plant, are given by herbalists for inflammation of the digestive system, inflamed joints, and skin problems. See p. 89.

DRIED RHIZOME

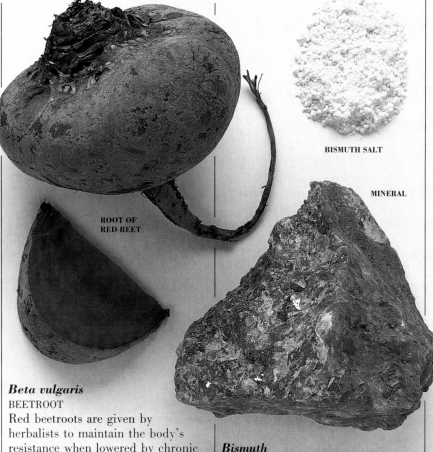

ROOT OF RED BEET

BISMUTH SALT

MINERAL

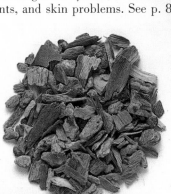

DRIED BARK

Beta vulgaris
BEETROOT
Red beetroots are given by herbalists to maintain the body's resistance when lowered by chronic infection. White beetroots are used against jaundice and liver damage caused by drug or alcohol abuse. In Europe, beetroot is taken as an anticancer treatment. See p. 89.

Bismuth
Salts of this common mineral are still frequently used in indigestion remedies and are now also given in orthodox medicine to encourage the healing of stomach ulcers. See p. 90.

Betula pendula
EUROPEAN WHITE BIRCH
The juice of birch leaves was said by Culpeper to be "good to wash sore mouths." Today, the silvery white bark and leaves are prescribed by herbalists for conditions such as arthritis, urinary tract infections, autoimmune disease, and fluid retention. See p. 90.

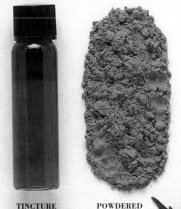

TINCTURE

POWDERED BARK

DRIED LEAVES

Berberis vulgaris
COMMON BARBERRY
Herbalists use tincture of barberry bark for liver ailments caused by alcohol or drug misuse. In Ayurvedic medicine, the herb is used against parasitic diseases and malaria, while Chinese physicians prescribe it for dysentery and diarrhea. See p. 89.

BRANCH

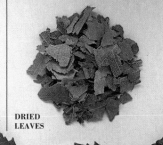

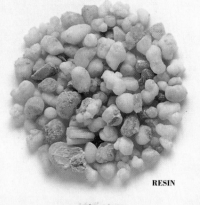

RESIN

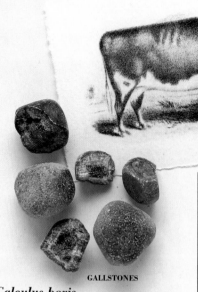

GALLSTONES

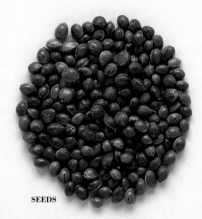

SEEDS

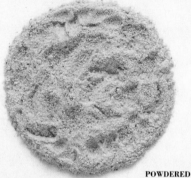

POWDERED RESIN

Boswellia thurifera
FRANKINCENSE
The resin of the frankincense tree has been used as an antiseptic by herbalists since before Christ. In Chinese medicine, it is given for ailments ranging from leprosy to coughs. See p. 90.

Calculus bovis
CATTLE GALLSTONES
The brittle bitter-tasting gallstones, or bezoars, that occur in many kinds of mammal have been used in traditional Eastern and Western medicine for centuries for fevers and other "hot" complaints. See p. 90.

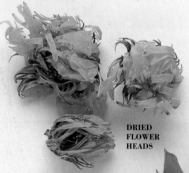

DRIED FLOWER HEADS

Cannabis sativa
MARIJUANA
Marijuana has a medical history in China and India of at least 1,500 years, and it is still used today in many systems of medicine. For example, the seeds are given by Chinese physicians as a tonic, laxative, and emollient. See p. 91.

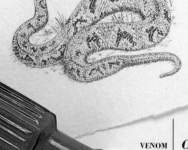

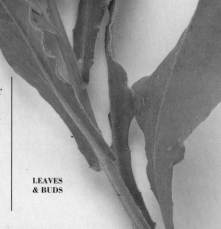

VENOM

Bothrops jararaca
PIT VIPER
Venom from this South American pit viper has two uses – to make an antidote for its bite, and as a source of the enzyme teprotide, which has been used to investigate high blood pressure. See p. 90.

Calendula officinalis
POT MARIGOLD
The flowers and leaves of the familiar garden marigold have been valued since antiquity for their range of actions, such as antiseptic and wound healing properties. They are used externally for leg ulcers, hemorrhoids, conjunctivitis, and eczema, and internally for ulcers and throat infections. See p. 91.

LEAVES & BUDS

CASSIA ACUTIFOLIA

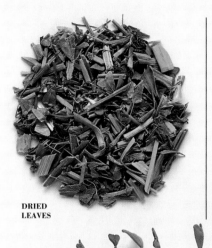

DRIED LEAVES

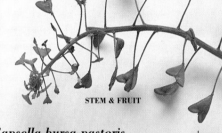

STEM & FRUIT

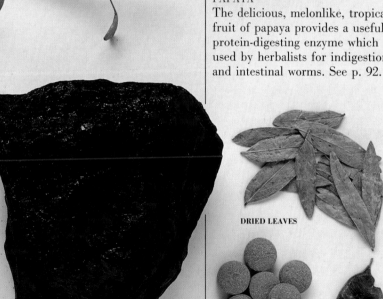

COAL

COAL TAR PASTE

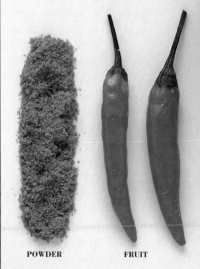

POWDER　　**FRUIT**

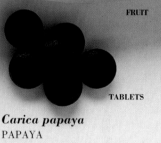

FRUIT

TABLETS

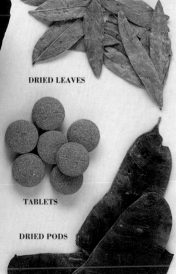

DRIED LEAVES

TABLETS

DRIED PODS

Capsella bursa-pastoris
SHEPHERD'S PURSE
A traditional medicine for stopping bleeding, shepherd's purse is still given by herbalists for many forms of bleeding, both internal and external, as well as for urinary tract problems. Its pale green hairy leaves are used to make infusions or tinctures. See p. 91.

Carica papaya
PAPAYA
The delicious, melonlike, tropical fruit of papaya provides a useful protein-digesting enzyme which is used by herbalists for indigestion and intestinal worms. See p. 92.

Capsicum
CHILE PEPPERS
The red or yellow fruit of these hot African and West Indian chiles is a popular aid for ailments that involve reduced blood circulation, such as poor digestion and chilblains (sores caused by exposure to extreme cold). See p. 91.

Carbon
COAL
Bituminous coal is the main kind of coal used as a medicinal source. Distilled, it gives rise to coal tar, which provides a common orthodox treatment for eczema, psoriasis, and dandruff. See p. 92.

Cassia acutifolia
ALEXANDRIAN SENNA
The pods and leaves of this small shrub provide one of the most widely used laxatives, an action first recorded by Arabian physicians. It is taken for constipation due to lack of bowel tone, but laxatives should not be overused. See p. 92.

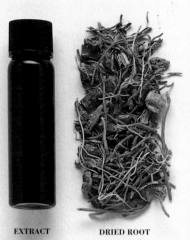

EXTRACT   **DRIED ROOT**

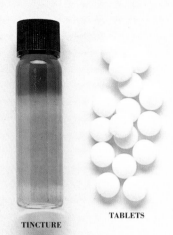

TINCTURE   **TABLETS**

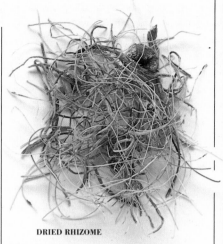

DRIED RHIZOME

Caulophyllum thalictroides
BLUE COHOSH
Native Americans introduced blue cohosh root to Europeans; they used it to ease the pain of childbirth. Herbalists still prescribe it for uterus problems such as menstrual cramps, as well as for rheumatism. See p. 92.

Cephaelis ipecacuanha
IPECACUANHA ROOT
Enthusiastically adopted from the New World by Europe in the 17th century, ipecacuanha root is used by herbalists and orthodox doctors for coughs and to cause vomiting after drug overdose. Homeopaths prescribe it for nausea and vomiting. See p. 92.

Chamaelirium luteum
RATTLESNAKE ROOT
The value of this rhizome in treating female reproductive disorders was learned from Native Americans. Herbalists still use it for such problems, including threatened miscarriage. See p. 93.

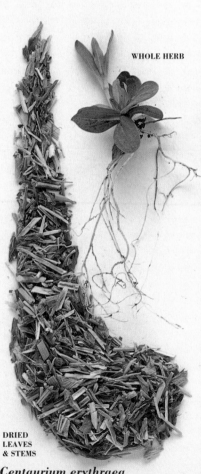

WHOLE HERB

DRIED LEAVES & STEMS

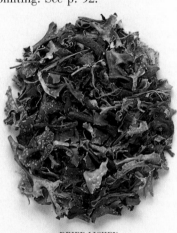

DRIED LICHEN

TABLETS

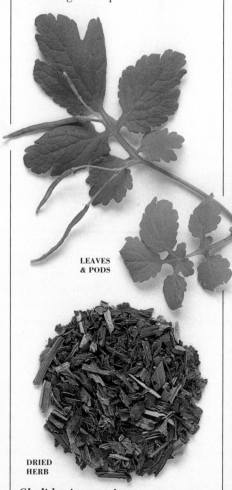

LEAVES & PODS

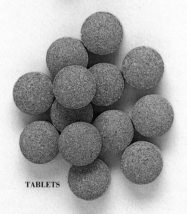

DRIED HERB

Centaurium erythraea
CENTAURY
The leaves and stems of centaury, which was named after a centaur who used it to cure a poisoned arrow wound, are now given by herbalists for digestive problems. See p. 92.

Cetraria islandica
ICELAND MOSS
This gray-brown or olive lichen of the cold north is given by herbalists to soothe the stomach, relieve vomiting, and help disperse phlegm. It is also included in proprietary cough medicines. See p. 93.

Chelidonium majus
GREATER CELANDINE
The whole herb, from its delicate bright yellow flowers to its pale green leaves, is used by homeopaths and herbalists, East and West, for a wide range of conditions, from jaundice to bronchitis. See p. 93.

CIMICIFUGA RACEMOSA

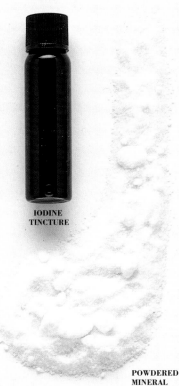

IODINE TINCTURE

POWDERED MINERAL

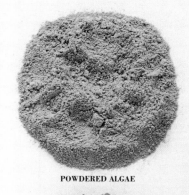

POWDERED ALGAE

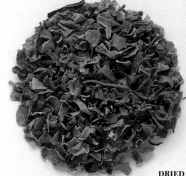

DRIED ALGAE

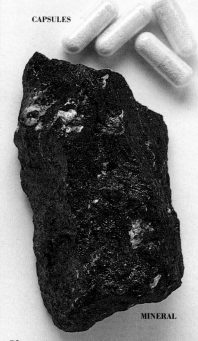

CAPSULES

MINERAL

Chili saltpeter
SALTPETER

This mineral is a main source of the essential mineral iodine, which is used in orthodox medicine to treat an overactive thyroid gland and in disinfectants. See p. 93.

Chondrus crispus
IRISH MOSS

This algae from the cool North Atlantic is dried and used by herbalists to soothe internal body surfaces, and as an emulsifier in medicines and foods. See p. 94.

Chromite
CHROMIUM ORE

This mineral is the only ore of chromium, a metal that is one of the most recently recognized essential nutrients. Studies have shown that chromium is important for insulin function. It is often lost in food-refining processes. See p. 94.

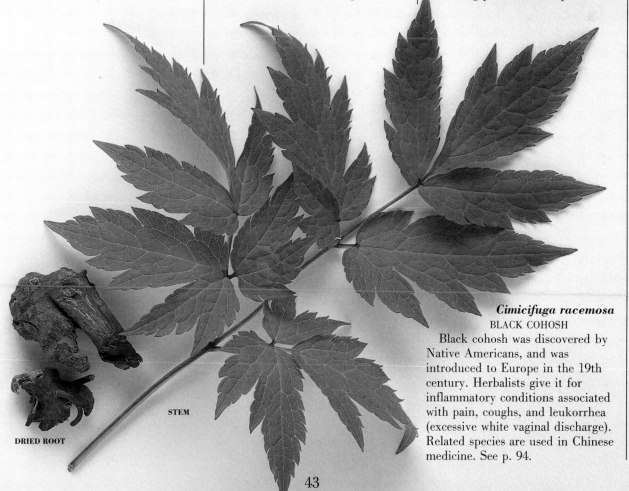

STEM

DRIED ROOT

Cimicifuga racemosa
BLACK COHOSH

Black cohosh was discovered by Native Americans, and was introduced to Europe in the 19th century. Herbalists give it for inflammatory conditions associated with pain, coughs, and leukorrhea (excessive white vaginal discharge). Related species are used in Chinese medicine. See p. 94.

CINCHONA SUCCIRUBRA

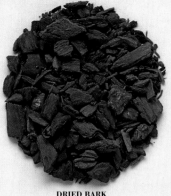

DRIED BARK

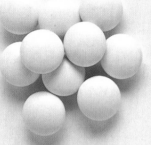

QUININE SULFATE TABLETS

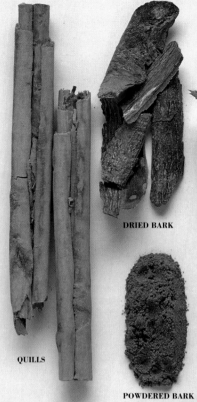

DRIED BARK

QUILLS

POWDERED BARK

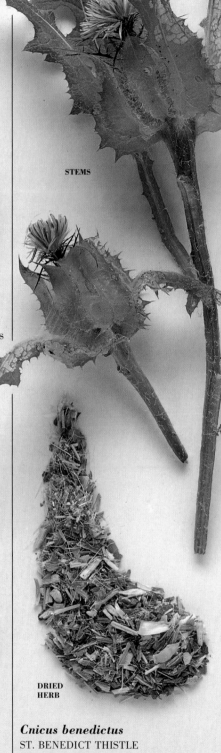

STEMS

DRIED HERB

Cinchona succirubra
PERUVIAN BARK
The Spanish invaders of South America first learnt of Peruvian bark's usefulness as a remedy for malaria from the indigenous peoples. The bark and extracted quinine are still widely used to prevent and treat malaria today See p. 94.

Cinnamomum zeylanicum
CINNAMON
The inner bark of this tropical tree's shoots is sold in rolled-up quills, dried, or powdered. Cinnamon has been valued in medicine for thousands of years for colds and flu, and digestive problems. See p. 95.

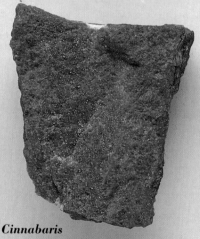

Cinnabaris
CINNABAR
The Romans were the first to extract mercury from this crimson ore. Mercury was a known poison, yet was commonly used in the West until 1900. Cinnabar is still prescribed in Chinese medicine, and mercury is used homeopathically and in tooth fillings. See p. 95.

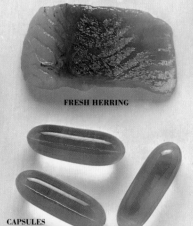

FRESH HERRING

CAPSULES

Clupeiformes species
HERRING FAMILY
Herring flesh is rich in essential fatty acids, which are thought to be protective against heart disease. Oil is extracted from the flesh and given in capsules in orthodox medicine to prevent arteriosclerosis (the clogging of arteries with cholesterol deposits). See p. 95.

Cnicus benedictus
ST. BENEDICT THISTLE
Named holy thistle because it was seen as a remedy for the plague, the flowering plant is used internally by herbalists for sluggish or disturbed digestion. Externally it is applied to wounds and ulcers. See p. 95.

CONCHA OSTREA

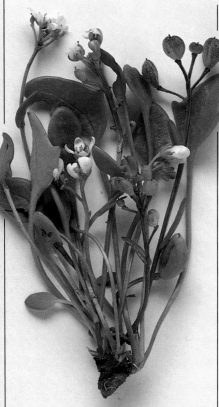

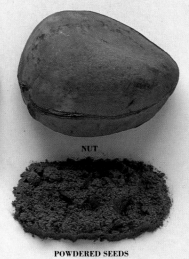

NUT

POWDERED SEEDS

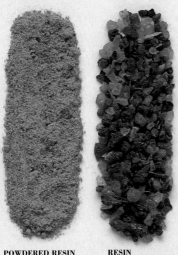

POWDERED RESIN   RESIN

Cola vera
COLA TREE

A favorite stimulant of people in West Africa, South America, and Asia, whole or powdered seeds from the nut are used to counter tiredness and stimulate appetite. See p. 96.

Commiphora molmol
MYRRH

One of the oldest known medicines, it is valued by herbalists for wounds and infections, and as a mouthwash. It is also used by Ayurvedic and Chinese physicians. See p. 96.

Cochlearia officinalis
SCURVY GRASS

Taken for scurvy long before the cause of the disease was discovered, scurvy grass is now known to be as rich in vitamin C as oranges. Today, herbalists apply the leaves to slow-healing wounds or ulcers. See p. 95.

POWDERED SHELL

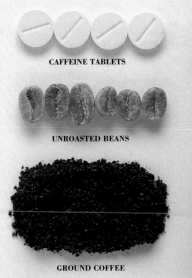

CAFFEINE TABLETS

UNROASTED BEANS

GROUND COFFEE

Coffea arabica
COFFEE

Coffee was introduced to Europe in the 17th century and has since been a commonly used stimulant. Given by herbalists for narcotic poisoning, it is also added to painkillers and is used homeopathically. See p. 96.

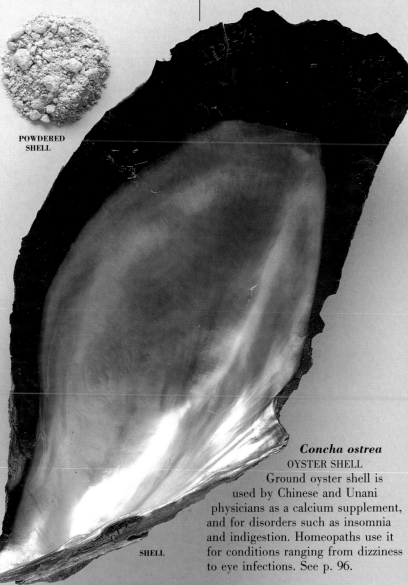

SHELL

Concha ostrea
OYSTER SHELL

Ground oyster shell is used by Chinese and Unani physicians as a calcium supplement, and for disorders such as insomnia and indigestion. Homeopaths use it for conditions ranging from dizziness to eye infections. See p. 96.

CONVALLARIA MAJALIS

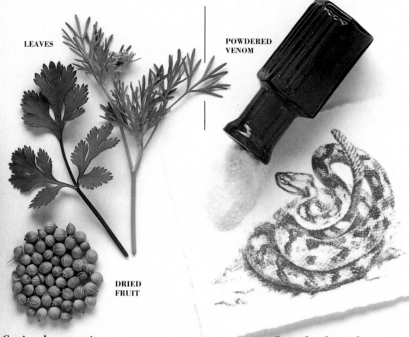

LEAVES

POWDERED VENOM

DRIED FRUIT

Coriandrum sativum
CORIANDER
Coriander fruits are used by
herbalists worldwide to relieve or
prevent gas and colic. Ayurvedic
medicine prescribes them for
conditions ranging from burns to
allergies, and Chinese medicine uses
them for stomachache, measles, and
nausea. See p. 97.

Crotalus horridus
RATTLESNAKE
Homeopaths use the venom from
this North American rattlesnake for
swelling and pain that is aggravated,
not relieved, by the application of
pressure. The snake gets its name
from the rattle made when the
horny rings of its tail vibrate as it
attacks. See p. 97.

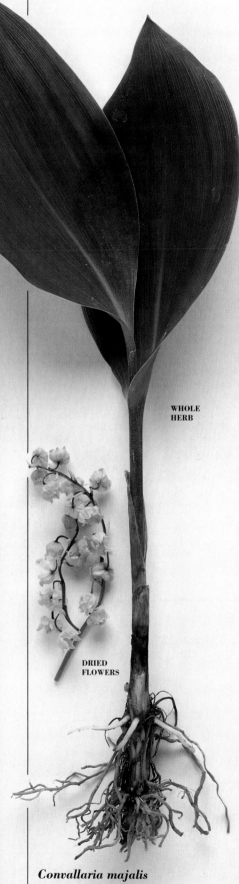

WHOLE HERB

DRIED FLOWERS

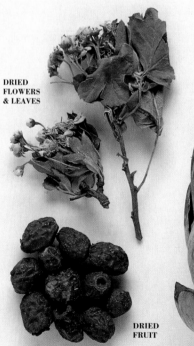

DRIED FLOWERS & LEAVES

DRIED FRUIT

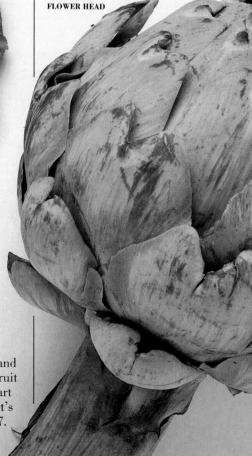

ARTICHOKE FLOWER HEAD

Convallaria majalis
LILY OF THE VALLEY
The flowering tops and root have a
similar, but safer, effect on the heart
to *Digitalis* (see p. 48) and are
given by herbalists for heart failure
and fluid retention. See p. 97.

Crataegus oxycanthoides
HAWTHORN
Given by herbalists, both East and
West, the flowers, leaves, and fruit
form one of the most useful heart
remedies, and improve the heart's
action and circulation. See p. 97.

DEMOSPONGIAE

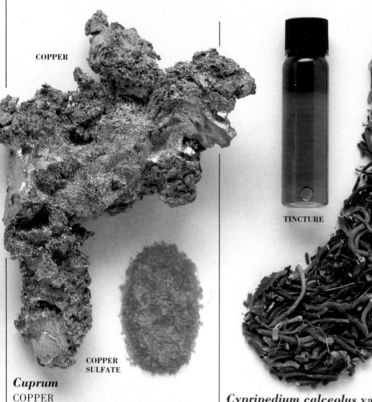

COPPER

COPPER
SULFATE

TINCTURE

DRIED
ROOT

INFUSION

DRIED
HERB

Cuprum
COPPER
Copper sulfate is given in orthodox medicine for copper deficiencies. Copper is also used in homeopathy and Chinese medicine. See p. 97.

Cypripedium calceolus var. pubescens
LARGE YELLOW LADY'S SLIPPER
This herb was passed on to Europe from the Native Americans, who knew of its root's sedative and relaxing powers. See p. 98.

Daucus carota
WILD CARROT
The whole herb, including the seeds and the feathery leaves, has been used medicinally since ancient Greek times. Today, herbalists and Ayurvedic physicians give it for urinary tract problems, colic, gout, and amenorrhea. See p. 98.

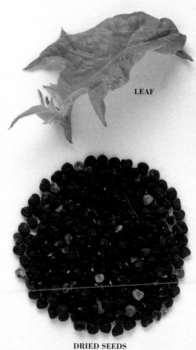

LEAF

DRIED SEEDS

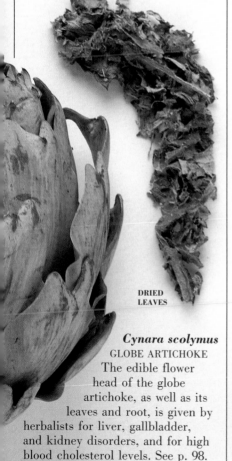

DRIED
LEAVES

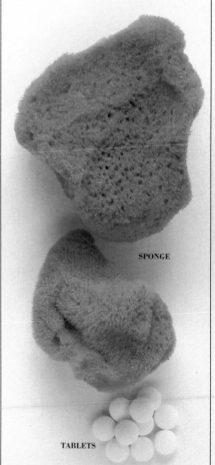

SPONGE

TABLETS

Cynara scolymus
GLOBE ARTICHOKE
The edible flower head of the globe artichoke, as well as its leaves and root, is given by herbalists for liver, gallbladder, and kidney disorders, and for high blood cholesterol levels. See p. 98.

Datura stramonium
JIMSONWEED
The leaves and seeds are dangerous for self-use, but are given by herbalists to relieve muscle spasms, for instance in asthma and Parkinson's disease. See p. 98.

Demospongiae
HORNY SPONGE
Burnt sponge is applied externally in Unani medicine for wounds and swellings, and to improve eyesight. Homeopaths give it in tablet form for swollen thyroid glands, headaches, and coughs. See p. 99.

DIGITALIS SPECIES

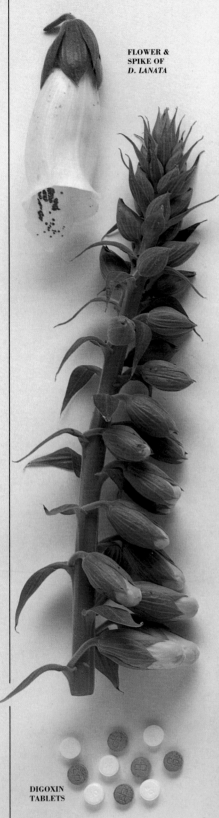

FLOWER &
SPIKE OF
D. LANATA

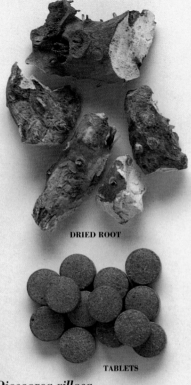

DRIED ROOT

TABLETS

Dioscorea villosa
WILD YAM
Wild yam root is used in the
preparation of steroids by the
pharmaceutical industry. Herbalists
use it for conditions ranging from
rheumatic diseases to ovarian pain.
See p. 99.

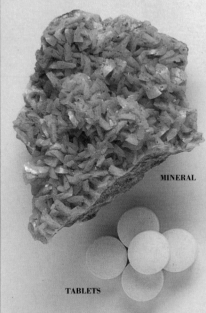

MINERAL

TABLETS

Dolomite
CALCIUM MAGNESIUM CARBONATE
Powdered dolomite is taken as a
supplement, providing calcium and
magnesium for people who want to
increase their intake. The crystals,
which originate from the shells of
tiny sea animals, are translucent and
colorless, white, or pink. See p. 99.

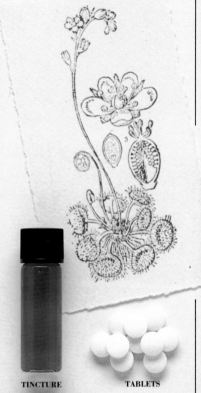

TINCTURE   TABLETS

Drosera rotundifolia
ROUND-LEAVED SUNDEW
This insect-catching plant is used in
its entirety by herbalists to relieve
bronchial spasm, for example in
asthma. Homeopaths give it for
coughs and sore throats. See p. 99.

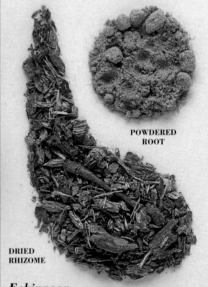

POWDERED
ROOT

DRIED
RHIZOME

Echinacea angustifolia
PURPLE CONEFLOWER
The roots and rhizome are being
studied as a possible treatment for
AIDS. Coneflower is also used by
herbalists as an antiviral remedy for
infections ranging from tonsillitis to
blood poisoning. See p. 100.

DIGOXIN
TABLETS

Digitalis purpurea & D. lanata ☠
FOXGLOVE
Until the late 18th century, the
value of foxglove leaves as a heart
remedy went unrecognized. Now,
extracted digoxin from *D. lanata* is
widely prescribed in orthodox
medicine for heart failure and
irregular heartbeat. See p. 99.

ERYTHROXYLUM COCA

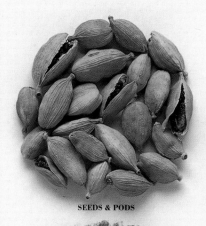

SEEDS & PODS

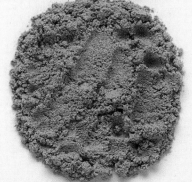

POWDERED SEEDS

Elettaria cardamomum
CARDAMOM
The seeds are given herbally for digestive problems. Ayurvedic and Chinese physicians also prescribe them. See p. 100.

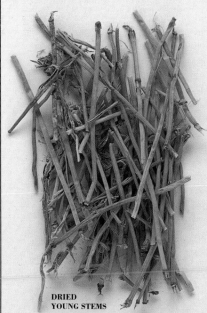

DRIED YOUNG STEMS

Ephedra sinica
MA HUANG
Given for asthma in China for 5,000 years, the young stems of this shrub were only established in Western medicine some 95 years ago as a source of ephedrine, a drug still prescribed for asthma. See p. 100.

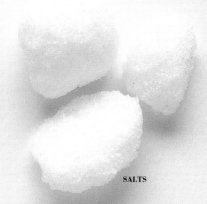

SALTS

Epsomite
EPSOM SALTS
Ground down to a salt, this mineral has been one of the most popular orthodox remedies for constipation and hangovers. However, overuse is not advisable. See p. 100.

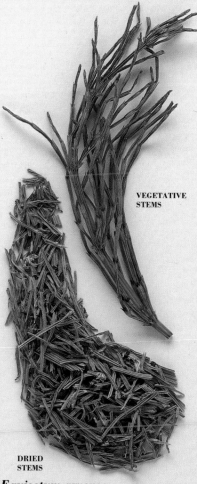

VEGETATIVE STEMS

DRIED STEMS

Equisetum arvense
HORSETAIL
The vegetative stems of horsetail are a long-established remedy given by herbalists for urinary and prostate conditions, and to help heal lung damage caused, for example, by tuberculosis. See p. 101.

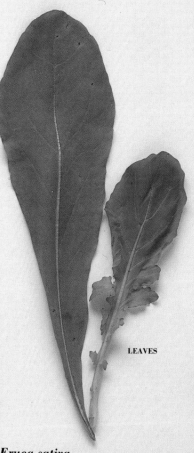

LEAVES

Eruca sativa
ROCKET
Rocket leaves are a popular salad ingredient, having a sharp, peppery taste. They have been used medicinally since Roman times and are now given by herbalists to help digestion and support the body's lymphatic system. See p. 101.

COCAINE POWDER

Erythroxylum coca
COCA
Coca leaves, chewed as a stimulant by Peruvians for centuries, have been used in orthodox medicine as a source of cocaine. This drug is now used mainly as a local anesthetic during minor surgery. See p. 101.

EUCALYPTUS GLOBULUS

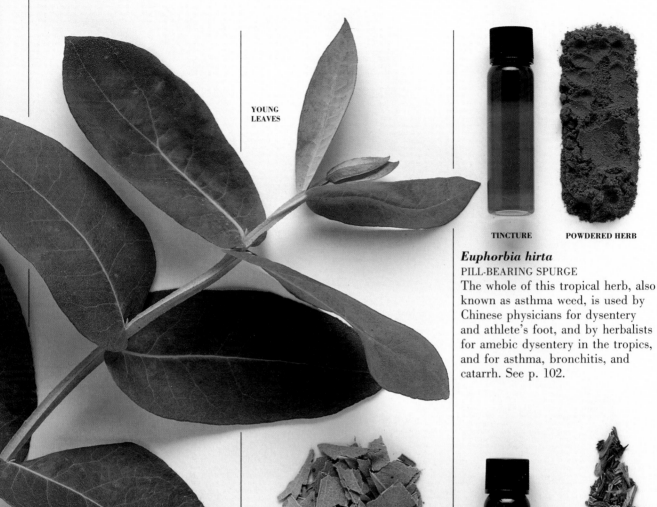

YOUNG
LEAVES

TINCTURE   POWDERED HERB

Euphorbia hirta
PILL-BEARING SPURGE
The whole of this tropical herb, also
known as asthma weed, is used by
Chinese physicians for dysentery
and athlete's foot, and by herbalists
for amebic dysentery in the tropics,
and for asthma, bronchitis, and
catarrh. See p. 102.

DRIED
LEAVES

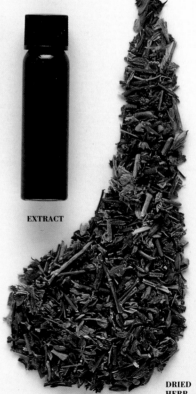

Eucalyptus globulus
BLUE GUM
This gum tree, like many Australian
gums, provides oil from its leaves
that is widely used in many forms
of medicine for coughs, colds, and
strained muscles. See p. 101.

EXTRACT

DRIED
HERB

LEAVES

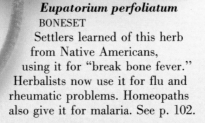

DRIED
HERB

Eupatorium perfoliatum
BONESET
Settlers learned of this herb
from Native Americans,
using it for "break bone fever."
Herbalists now use it for flu and
rheumatic problems. Homeopaths
also give it for malaria. See p. 102.

Euphrasia officinalis
EYEBRIGHT
Eyebright's flower looks like a
bloodshot eye, which encouraged
use of the herb for eye ailments.
Herbalists still give it for sinusitis
and conjunctivitis, and homeopaths
use it for hay fever. See p. 102.

*F*LUORITE

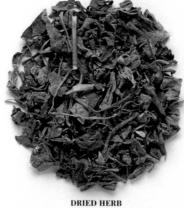

GRAIN

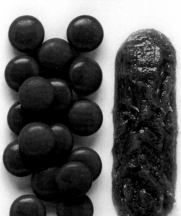

DRIED HERB

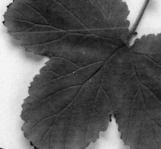

DRIED HERB

Fagopyrum esculentum
BUCKWHEAT
The leaves are used for conditions ranging from high blood pressure to frostbite. Chinese doctors give buckwheat for bites, stings, trauma, and menstrual cramps. See p. 102.

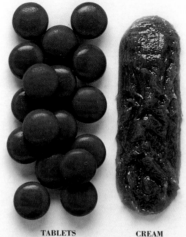

TABLETS   CREAM

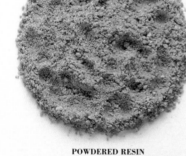

POWDERED RESIN

Ferula assa-foetida
ASAFETIDA
Resin from the root, also named devil's dung because of its nasty smell, is given by herbalists for colic, indigestion, bronchitis, and irritability. Ayurvedic uses are similar. See p. 102.

Ficaria ranunculoides
PILEWORT
The common name of pilewort reflects the shape of its tubers, which look like hemorrhoids, and its use. It is given internally as tablets and externally as a cream for hemorrhoids. See p. 103.

DRIED STEMS

LEAF

Filipendula ulmaria
MEADOWSWEET
The herb is used whole as a painkiller and for problems of digestion, such as peptic ulceration. See p. 103.

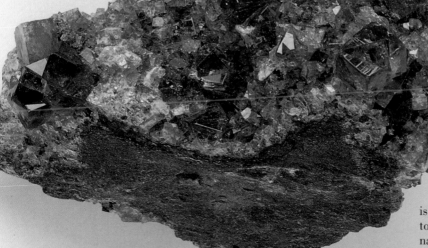

Fluorite
CALCIUM FLUORIDE
The main source of fluorine, an essential mineral variably supplied by food and water, calcium fluoride is given to increase resistance to tooth decay. Fluorite is used in its natural form in Chinese and homeopathic medicine. See p. 103.

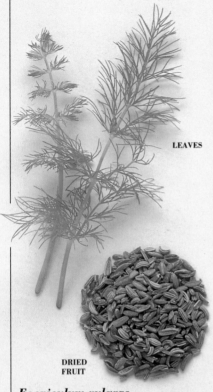

LEAVES

DRIED
FRUIT

Foeniculum vulgare
FENNEL
The seeds and root from this herb
have long been valued by cooks and
herbalists, both East and West, to
prevent and treat indigestion, gas,
and colic. See p. 103.

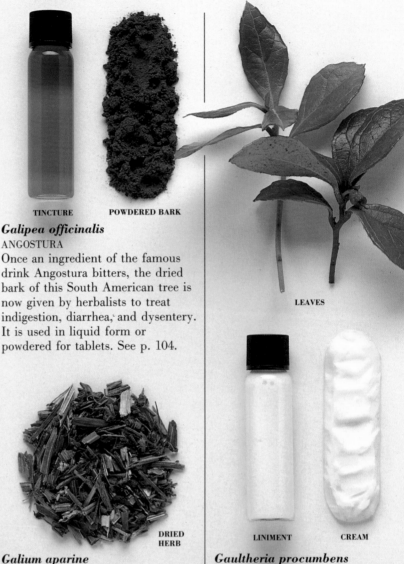

TINCTURE   POWDERED BARK

Galipea officinalis
ANGOSTURA
Once an ingredient of the famous
drink Angostura bitters, the dried
bark of this South American tree is
now given by herbalists to treat
indigestion, diarrhea, and dysentery.
It is used in liquid form or
powdered for tablets. See p. 104.

DRIED
HERB

Galium aparine
CLEAVERS
A popular "spring-cleansing" tonic,
cleavers has been used for centuries
to purify the blood and treat skin
diseases. The whole herb is now
given by herbalists for eczematous
rashes, swollen lymph glands, and
urinary tract problems. See p. 104.

LEAVES

LINIMENT   CREAM

Gaultheria procumbens
WINTERGREEN
The leaves of this North American
shrub are used by herbalists to
relieve the pain of rheumatism,
sprains, and sciatica. Synthetic oil of
wintergreen is sold over the counter
as a liniment or cream for similar
uses. See p. 104.

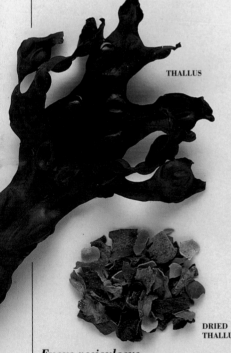

THALLUS

DRIED
THALLUS

Fucus vesiculosus
BLADDERWRACK
High in iodine content, this seaweed
is used by herbalists to treat an
underactive thyroid gland and
related obesity. Applied externally it
is antirheumatic. See p. 104.

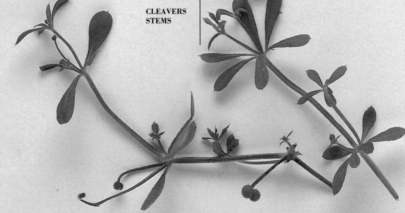

CLEAVERS
STEMS

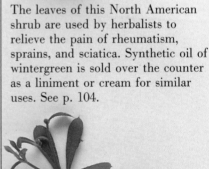

GLYCYRRHIZA GLABRA

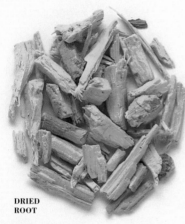

DRIED ROOT

Gelsemium sempervirens ☠
YELLOW JESSAMINE
Also known as false jasmine, it is not actually a jasmine. The root is given externally by herbalists for toothache, but, as it is poisonous, it is used internally only in homeopathic doses. See p. 104.

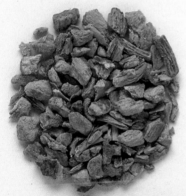

DRIED ROOT

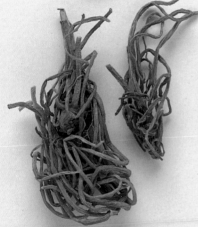

DRIED CHINESE GENTIAN ROOT

Gentiana lutea
YELLOW GENTIAN
The root of this bitter-tasting alpine plant is given by herbalists for digestive problems from anorexia to hepatitis. Chinese medicine uses *Gentiana* species for eye and skin problems. Some over-the-counter tonics contain gentian. See p. 105.

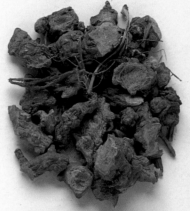

DRIED RHIZOME

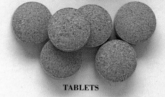

TABLETS

Geranium maculatum
WILD GERANIUM
The rhizome, originally used by Native Americans as an astringent, is now given internally by herbalists for stomach disturbances such as diarrhea, food poisoning, and peptic ulcers. See p. 105.

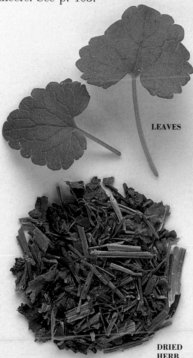

LEAVES

DRIED HERB

Glechoma hederacea
GROUND IVY
This herb is valued by herbalists for ailments as varied as catarrh, hemorrhoids, bronchitis, cystitis, and indigestion. Chinese physicians prescribe it for flu, kidney stones, traumatic injuries, rheumatoid arthritis, and skin sores. See p. 105.

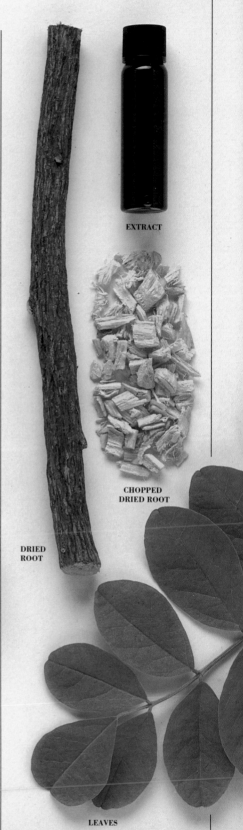

EXTRACT

CHOPPED DRIED ROOT

DRIED ROOT

LEAVES

Glycyrrhiza glabra
LICORICE
One of the most used medicines of the ancient world, the root is still given by herbalists for peptic ulcers, bronchitis, and rheumatism. Chinese medicine prescribes it for similar complaints. Orthodox medicine gives extracts for peptic ulcers. See p. 105.

GRAPHITE

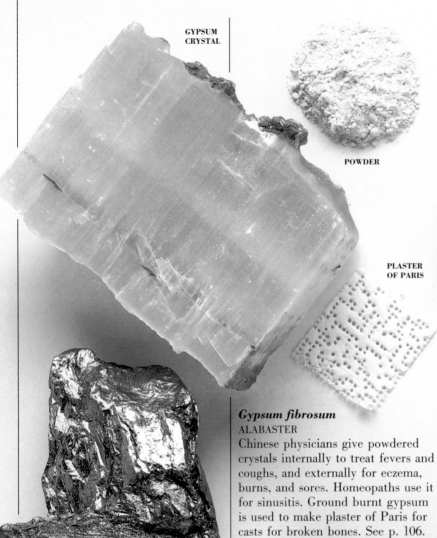

GYPSUM CRYSTAL

POWDER

PLASTER OF PARIS

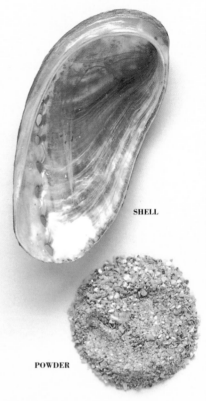

SHELL

POWDER

Gypsum fibrosum
ALABASTER
Chinese physicians give powdered crystals internally to treat fevers and coughs, and externally for eczema, burns, and sores. Homeopaths use it for sinusitis. Ground burnt gypsum is used to make plaster of Paris for casts for broken bones. See p. 106.

Haliotis gigantea
ABALONE
Ear-shaped abalone shells are prescribed in Chinese medicine for many conditions, including fevers, aches, dizziness, red eyes, and blurred vision. See p. 106.

Graphite
BLACK LEAD
This dark gray form of carbon, familiar in pencils, is a key homeopathic remedy for skin ailments, including psoriasis, eczema, and cracked and weeping skin. It is also given by homeopaths for menstrual problems. See p. 105.

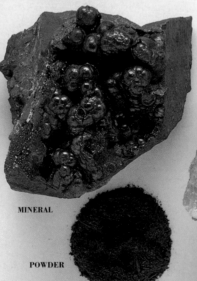

MINERAL

POWDER

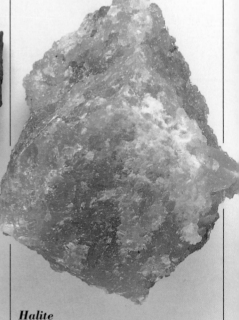

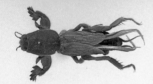

Gryllotalpa orientalis
MOLE-CRICKET
The bodies of male mole-crickets – earth-tunneling relatives of the cricket – are given in Chinese medicine for water retention, to ripen boils and abscesses, and for difficult labor. See p. 106.

Haematitum
HEMATITE
This naturally occurring iron ore, in the form mixed with red clay, is given by Chinese doctors for a range of symptoms, including biliousness, dizziness, headaches, hiccups, and nausea and vomiting. See p. 106.

Halite
ROCK SALT
Rock salt is used homeopathically for sneezing, colds, eczema, hives, thrush, menstrual problems, and migraines. In Ayurvedic medicine it is given for digestive problems. See p. 106.

HIPPOCAMPUS KELLOGGI

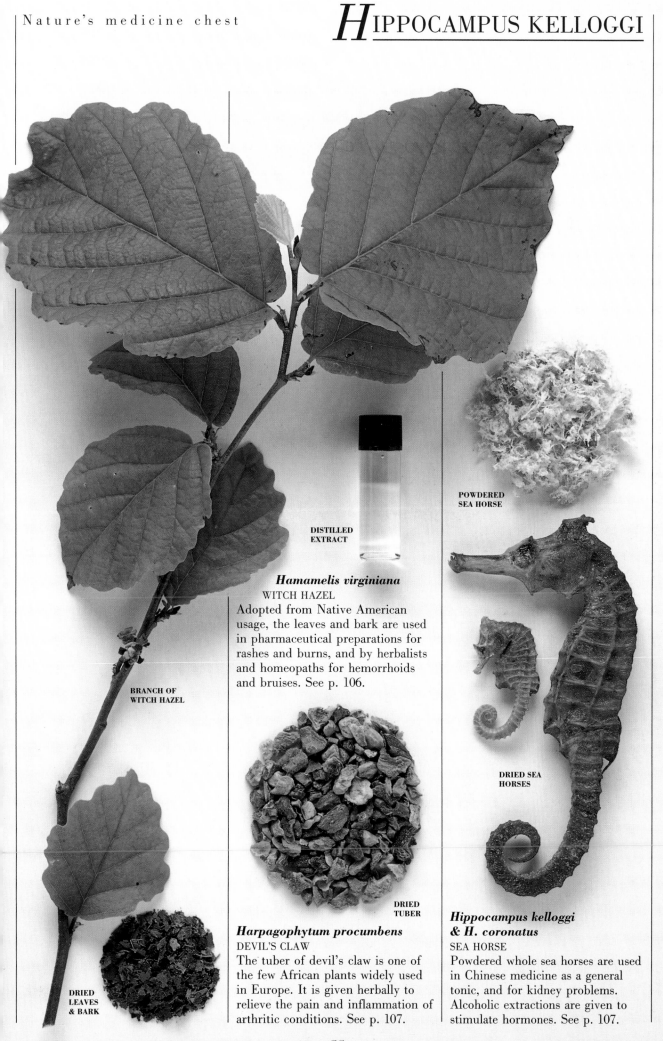

DISTILLED EXTRACT

POWDERED SEA HORSE

Hamamelis virginiana
WITCH HAZEL
Adopted from Native American usage, the leaves and bark are used in pharmaceutical preparations for rashes and burns, and by herbalists and homeopaths for hemorrhoids and bruises. See p. 106.

BRANCH OF WITCH HAZEL

DRIED SEA HORSES

DRIED TUBER

DRIED LEAVES & BARK

Harpagophytum procumbens
DEVIL'S CLAW
The tuber of devil's claw is one of the few African plants widely used in Europe. It is given herbally to relieve the pain and inflammation of arthritic conditions. See p. 107.

Hippocampus kelloggi & H. coronatus
SEA HORSE
Powdered whole sea horses are used in Chinese medicine as a general tonic, and for kidney problems. Alcoholic extractions are given to stimulate hormones. See p. 107.

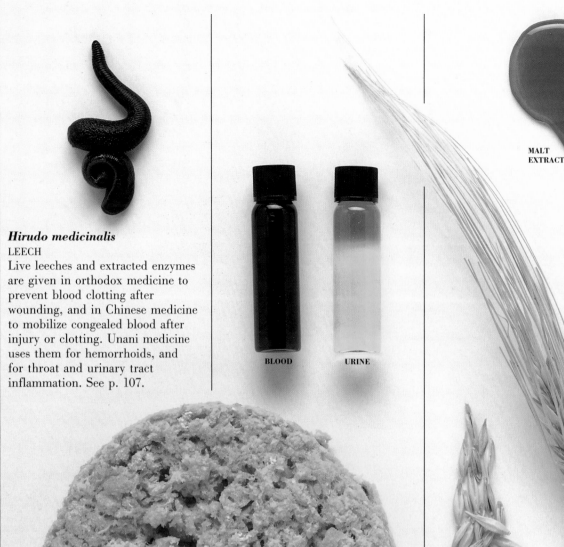

Hirudo medicinalis
LEECH
Live leeches and extracted enzymes are given in orthodox medicine to prevent blood clotting after wounding, and in Chinese medicine to mobilize congealed blood after injury or clotting. Unani medicine uses them for hemorrhoids, and for throat and urinary tract inflammation. See p. 107.

BLOOD

URINE

MALT
EXTRACT

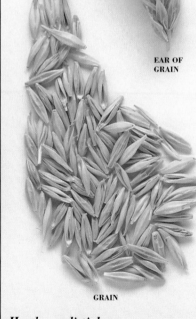

EAR OF
GRAIN

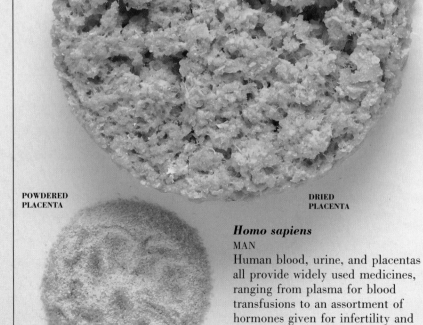

POWDERED
PLACENTA

DRIED
PLACENTA

GRAIN

Homo sapiens
MAN
Human blood, urine, and placentas all provide widely used medicines, ranging from plasma for blood transfusions to an assortment of hormones given for infertility and other conditions. Chinese medicine prescribes dried placenta as a tonic and for impotence. See p. 107.

Hordeum distichon
BARLEY
Traditionally, barley grain (polished or germinating) is used as a convalescent food in forms such as soup, malt extract, or barley water, especially after diarrhea or bowel disease. Chinese physicians use it for loss of appetite, poor digestion, and bloating. See p. 108.

HYPERICUM PERFORATUM

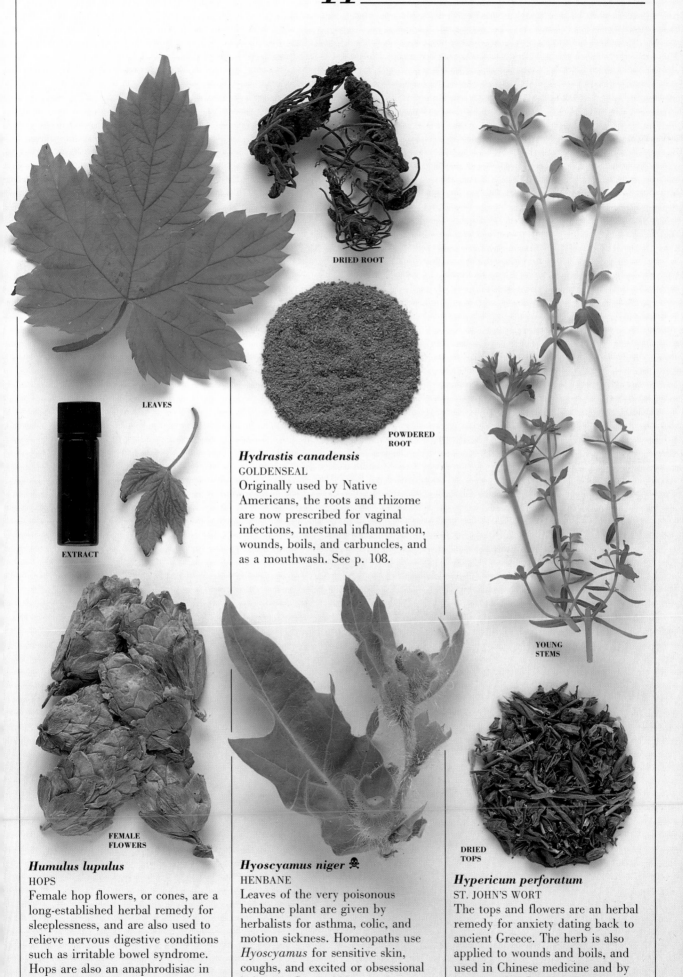

DRIED ROOT

LEAVES

POWDERED ROOT

EXTRACT

YOUNG STEMS

FEMALE FLOWERS

DRIED TOPS

Hydrastis canadensis
GOLDENSEAL
Originally used by Native Americans, the roots and rhizome are now prescribed for vaginal infections, intestinal inflammation, wounds, boils, and carbuncles, and as a mouthwash. See p. 108.

Humulus lupulus
HOPS
Female hop flowers, or cones, are a long-established herbal remedy for sleeplessness, and are also used to relieve nervous digestive conditions such as irritable bowel syndrome. Hops are also an anaphrodisiac in men. See p. 108.

Hyoscyamus niger ☠
HENBANE
Leaves of the very poisonous henbane plant are given by herbalists for asthma, colic, and motion sickness. Homeopaths use *Hyoscyamus* for sensitive skin, coughs, and excited or obsessional behavior. See p. 109.

Hypericum perforatum
ST. JOHN'S WORT
The tops and flowers are an herbal remedy for anxiety dating back to ancient Greece. The herb is also applied to wounds and boils, and used in Chinese medicine and by homeopaths. See p. 109.

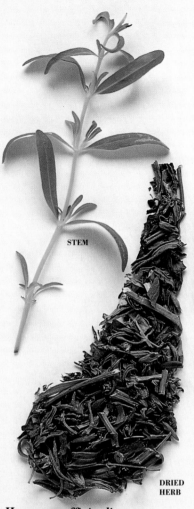

STEM

DRIED
HERB

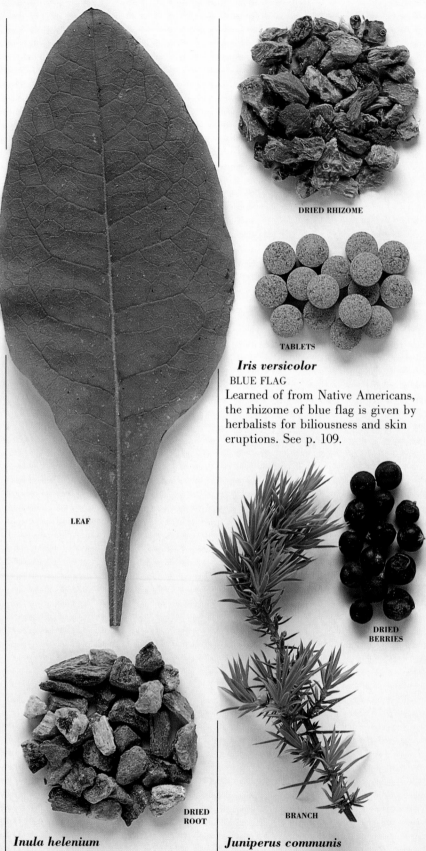

LEAF

DRIED
RHIZOME

TABLETS

Iris versicolor
BLUE FLAG
Learned of from Native Americans,
the rhizome of blue flag is given by
herbalists for biliousness and skin
eruptions. See p. 109.

DRIED
BERRIES

Hyssopus officinalis
HYSSOP
Herbalists give the whole herb for
bronchitis, chronic nasal catarrh,
coughs, and colds. Giant hyssop is
used in Chinese medicine for
vomiting, wounds, diarrhea, and
angina. See p. 109.

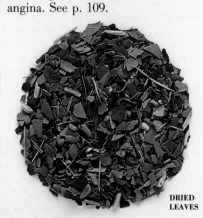

DRIED
LEAVES

DRIED
ROOT

BRANCH

Ilex paraguariensis
YERBA MATÉ
The caffeine-rich leaves of this South
American tree, used locally as a
stimulant and appetite suppressant,
have become a herbal remedy for
nervous headache with fatigue and
to suppress the appetite. See p. 109.

Inula helenium
ELECAMPANE
This herb has long been grown in
European gardens as a medicine, and
is still given by herbalists for
respiratory conditions. Chinese
medicine uses it for similar purposes,
and for worms. See p. 109.

Juniperus communis
JUNIPER
Familiar as a flavoring of gin, the
berries of this evergreen tree have
been used to treat rheumatism,
colic, and infections of the urinary
tract since the time of the ancient
Greeks. See p. 110.

LAVANDULA ANGUSTIFOLIA

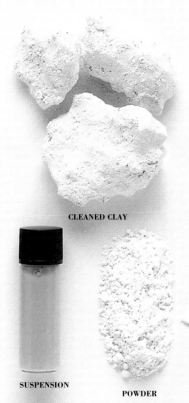

CLEANED CLAY

SUSPENSION

POWDER

Kaolin
HYDRATED ALUMINUM SILCATE
A fine white clay used internally in orthodox medicine for diarrhea and externally to reduce swelling and pain. It is also the base for many medical dusting powders. See p. 110.

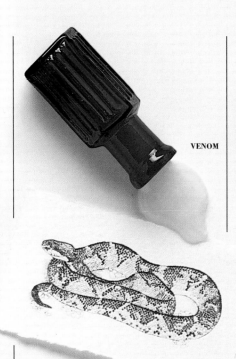

VENOM

Lachesis mutus
BUSHMASTER SURUCUCU SNAKE
The venom of this snake is given as a homeopathic remedy for headaches, palpitations, epilepsy, appendicitis, sore throats, boils, and menstrual cramps, particularly if the symptoms are on the left side of the body. See p. 110.

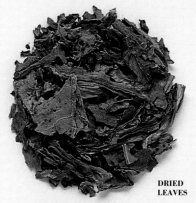

DRIED LEAVES

Lactuca virosa
WILD LETTUCE
The milky fluid from this herb is a mild sedative. Herbalists use the dried leaves for bronchitis, irritable coughs, restlessness, insomnia, and anxiety. See p. 111.

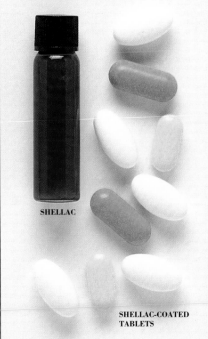

SHELLAC

SHELLAC-COATED TABLETS

Laccifer lacca
SHELLAC
A reddish resin exuded by female lac-insects, shellac is used in orthodox medicine to coat tablets, in Chinese medicine for bleeding, and by Unani physicians for blood, liver, and kidney disorders. See p. 110.

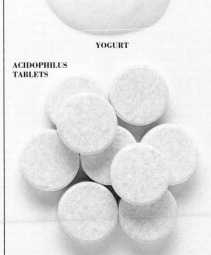

YOGURT

ACIDOPHILUS TABLETS

Lactobacillus acidophilus & Streptococcus thermophilus
YOGURT CULTURES
This is used in folk medicine and by some orthodox doctors to restore the microbial balance of the intestines when damaged by diarrhea or antibiotic drugs. See p. 110.

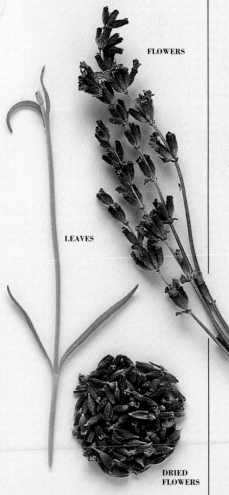

FLOWERS

LEAVES

DRIED FLOWERS

Lavandula angustifolia
LAVENDER
Lavender flowers have been used medicinally since Roman times. Herbalists now give lavender as a general relaxant and apply it externally to treat muscular pains and tension headaches. See p. 111.

LEONURUS CARDIACA

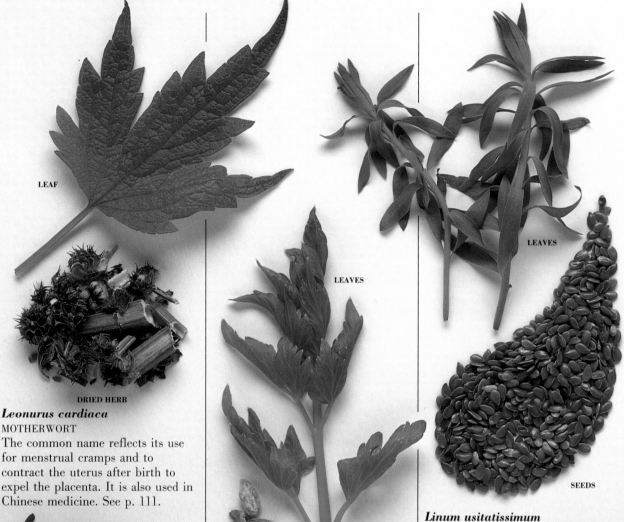

LEAF

DRIED HERB

LEAVES

LEAVES

SEEDS

DRIED ROOT

DRIED ROOT

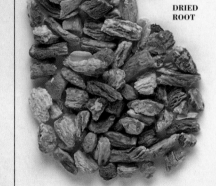

Leonurus cardiaca
MOTHERWORT
The common name reflects its use for menstrual cramps and to contract the uterus after birth to expel the placenta. It is also used in Chinese medicine. See p. 111.

Linum usitatissimum
LINSEED
Linseed seeds, from the flax plant that provides linen, are rich in polyunsaturated oils. Herbalists give them for some forms of constipation and coughs, and in a poultice to draw boils. See p. 112.

POWDERED ROOT

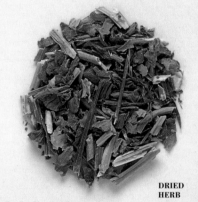

DRIED HERB

Leptandra virginica
BLACK ROOT
Learned of from Native Americans, use of the dried root spread to herbal medicine, which uses it as a laxative when there are liver or gallbladder problems. See p. 111.

Levisticum officinale
LOVAGE
Lovage root has a long medicinal history and is still given herbally for colicky indigestion, flatulence, bronchial infections, and menstrual problems. See p. 111.

Lobelia inflata
INDIAN TOBACCO
One of the key herbs of early Native American medicine, dried *Lobelia* is given herbally for asthma, chronic bronchitis, and rheumatic and muscular problems. It also alleviates nicotine withdrawal. See p. 112.

DRIED FLOWERS

LEAVES

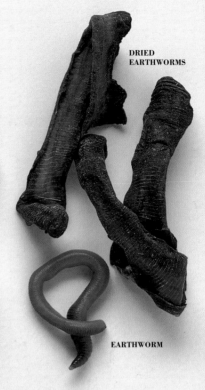

DRIED EARTHWORMS

EARTHWORM

Lonicera caprifolium
ITALIAN WOODBINE
Used as a remedy since Roman times, the flowers and leaves (berries are poisonous) are given by herbalists to encourage the coughing up of phlegm and as a mild laxative, and by Chinese physicians for colds, laryngitis, dysentery, food poisoning, rheumatism, and boils. See p. 112.

Lumbricum terrestris
EARTHWORM
Powdered dried earthworm is prescribed in Chinese medicine for the treatment of fevers, especially those related to the lungs, as an antidote to poisons, for breathing difficulties and coughs, and for excess water retention. See p. 112.

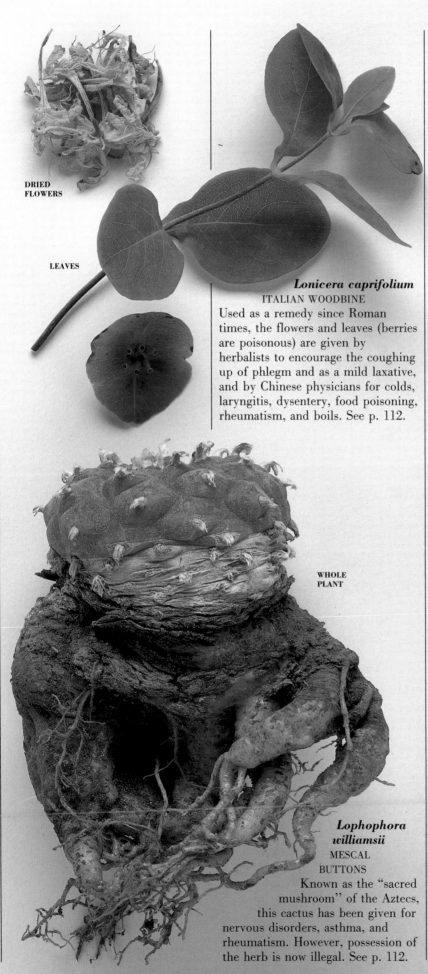

WHOLE PLANT

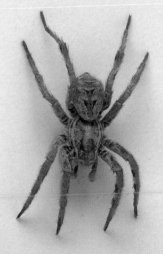

Lophophora williamsii
MESCAL BUTTONS
Known as the "sacred mushroom" of the Aztecs, this cactus has been given for nervous disorders, asthma, and rheumatism. However, possession of the herb is now illegal. See p. 112.

Lycosa cubensis
WOLF SPIDER
The wolf spider, though sometimes called a tarantula, comes from an entirely different family of spiders. Homeopaths use this species for swellings and abscesses. See p. 113.

LYTTA VESICATORIA

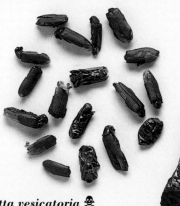

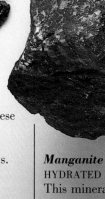

Lytta vesicatoria ☠
SPANISH FLY
Although lethally poisonous, these beetles can be used safely in homeopathic doses for local irritations and urinary infections. Chinese and Unani physicians mainly use them externally to improve circulation. See p. 113.

Manganite
HYDRATED MANGANESE OXIDE
This mineral is a source of manganese, a mineral essential to normal development and health. Although its actions in the body are little understood, supplements are given by some therapists to patients suffering from schizophrenia and diabetes. See p. 113.

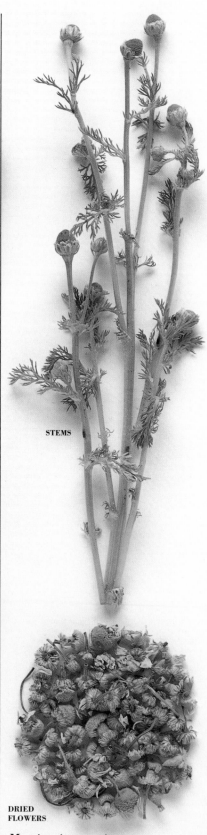

STEMS

MINERAL

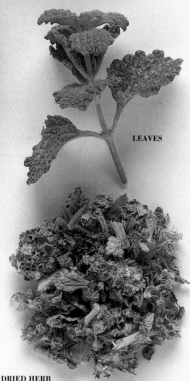

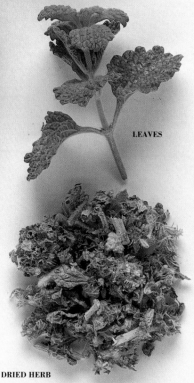

LEAVES

POWDER

DRIED HERB

DRIED FLOWERS

Magnetitum
MAGNETITE
An important ore of iron, it is naturally magnetic. The mineral is prescribed in Chinese medicine for tremors, palpitations, dizziness, blurred vision, vertigo, and asthma. See p. 113.

Marrubium vulgare
WHITE HOREHOUND
The whole herb has been given for coughs, catarrhal colds, and bronchitis since Egyptian times. It is also one of the bitter herbs eaten at Passover and is given by herbalists for poor digestion. See p. 113.

Matricaria recutita
GERMAN CHAMOMILE
The flowers are used by herbalists and homeopaths for many conditions, ranging from a nervous stomach and anxiety to teething and menstrual cramps. It is also applied externally for eczema. See p. 114.

Mirabilitum

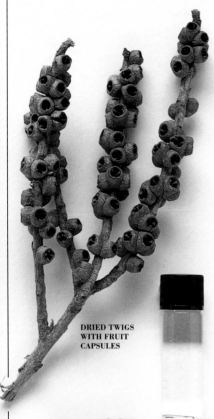

DRIED TWIGS
WITH FRUIT
CAPSULES

ESSENTIAL
OIL

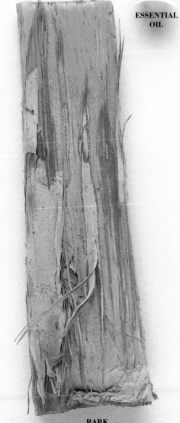

BARK

Melaleuca leucadendron
CAJEPUT
The twigs and fresh leaves of
cajeput, an Australian bottlebrush
tree, are given by herbalists to
relieve blocked sinuses, catarrh,
asthma, toothache, headaches, and
colic. See p. 114.

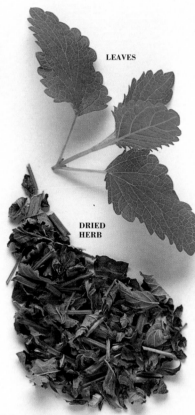

LEAVES

DRIED
HERB

Melissa officinalis
LEMON BALM
Named for its reputation as a
soother, lemon balm is a favorite
calming herb for anxiety and
nervous tension. See p. 114.

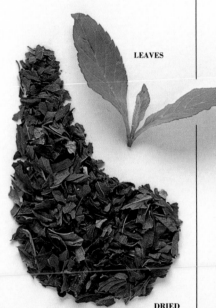

LEAVES

DRIED
HERB

Mentha x piperita
PEPPERMINT
Peppermint is the most widely used
herbal remedy in the Western
world. Herbalists use its digestion-
calming effect for colic, irritable
bowel syndrome, flatulence, and
morning sickness. See p. 114.

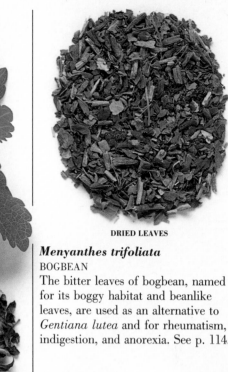

DRIED LEAVES

Menyanthes trifoliata
BOGBEAN
The bitter leaves of bogbean, named
for its boggy habitat and beanlike
leaves, are used as an alternative to
Gentiana lutea and for rheumatism,
indigestion, and anorexia. See p. 114.

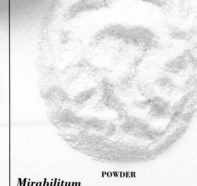

CRYSTALS

POWDER

Mirabilitum
GLAUBER'S SALT
Called the "wonder salt" by Dr.
Glauber, who developed its use as a
purgative, it is still used for
constipation in Chinese and
orthodox medicine but only for
robust patients. See p. 115.

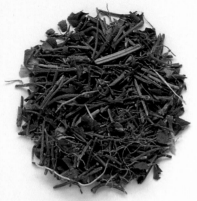

DRIED HERB

Mitchella repens
PARTRIDGEBERRY
Taken by Native American women
to make childbirth easier, it is still
given by herbalists to ease labor or
menstrual cramps, and for
exhaustion or irritability. See p. 115.

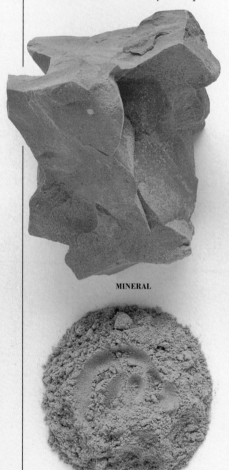

MINERAL

POWDER

Montmorillonite
FULLER'S EARTH
With silica, this soft rock makes
fuller's earth, so called because of its
use to cleanse and thicken cloth.
The powdered mineral is made into
dusting powders and given to absorb
harmful substances after poisoning.
See p. 115.

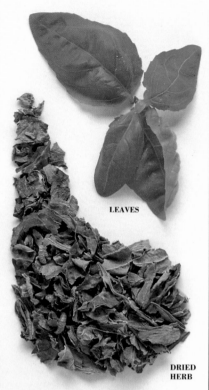

LEAVES

DRIED
HERB

Ocimum basilicum
SWEET BASIL
Sweet basil's use as a wonderful
flavor in food is matched by its
value as a digestive aid. Its volatile
oil is also applied externally in
herbal medicine as a treatment for
acne. See p. 115.

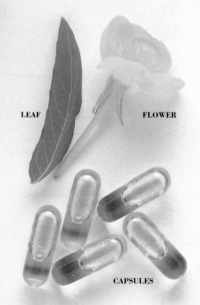

LEAF   FLOWER

CAPSULES

Oenothera biennis
EVENING PRIMROSE
Evening primrose oil is one of the
most researched plant remedies,
now an accepted treatment for
eczema, premenstrual syndrome,
and blood clot prevention. The
leaves have been used as a poultice
on boils and abscesses. See p. 115.

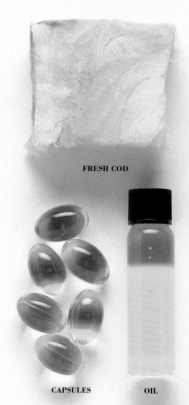

FRESH COD

CAPSULES   OIL

Oleum jacoris aselli
COD LIVER OIL
Cod liver oil, long used as a source
of vitamins A and D, is now being
validated in medical trials as a
treatment for eczema and arthritis,
for which it has long been used
traditionally. See p. 116.

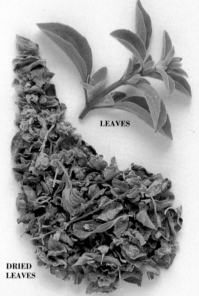

LEAVES

DRIED
LEAVES

Origanum marjorana
SWEET MARJORAM
The leaves of sweet marjoram,
closely related to oregano, are a
familiar culinary herb also used
herbally as a gentle carminative to
relieve gas and colic. It is also used
to make a digestive tea in Greece,
known as ditany. See p. 116.

PAEONIA OFFICINALIS

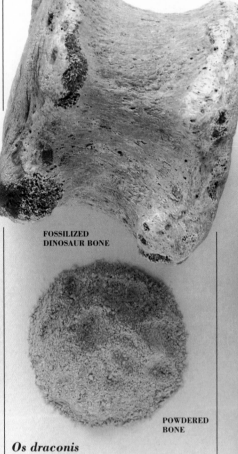

FOSSILIZED DINOSAUR BONE

POWDERED BONE

ROOT

LEAF & SEED HEAD

DRIED PETALS

DRIED ROOT

Os draconis
DRAGON BONES
Bones that have been fossilized over millions of years are called dragon bones by the Chinese. They are prescribed for nervous complaints, liver problems, and excessive body discharges. See p. 116.

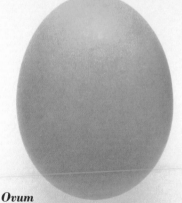

Ovum
HEN'S EGG
The yolk, white, and shell of a hen's egg are used in Chinese and Unani medicine for a wide range of complaints. Use of the yolk for heart conditions is echoed in the Western use of lecithin to break down blood fat deposits. See p. 116.

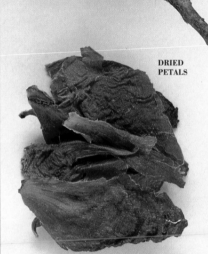

Paeonia officinalis
PEONY
The root and petals were used by herbalists to treat convulsions. Homeopaths give *Paeonia* for itching. Two related peonies are used for vascular problems, headaches, and stomach and menstrual cramps. See p. 116.

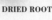

PANAX GINSENG

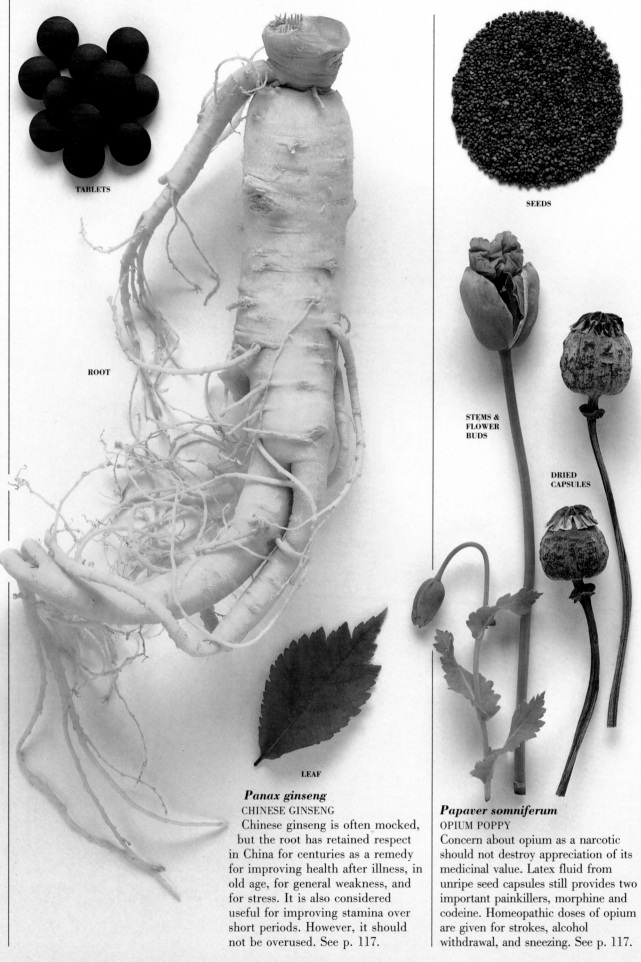

TABLETS

ROOT

LEAF

SEEDS

STEMS & FLOWER BUDS

DRIED CAPSULES

Panax ginseng
CHINESE GINSENG

Chinese ginseng is often mocked, but the root has retained respect in China for centuries as a remedy for improving health after illness, in old age, for general weakness, and for stress. It is also considered useful for improving stamina over short periods. However, it should not be overused. See p. 117.

Papaver somniferum
OPIUM POPPY

Concern about opium as a narcotic should not destroy appreciation of its medicinal value. Latex fluid from unripe seed capsules still provides two important painkillers, morphine and codeine. Homeopathic doses of opium are given for strokes, alcohol withdrawal, and sneezing. See p. 117.

66

PHYTOLACCA DECANDRA

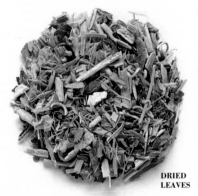

DRIED
LEAVES

Passiflora incarnata

PASSIONFLOWER

Passionflower, so called after the resemblance of the "crown" in its flower to Christ's crown of thorns, is given by herbalists to treat insomnia, restlessness, and irritability, and to relieve muscle spasms associated with nerves. See p. 117.

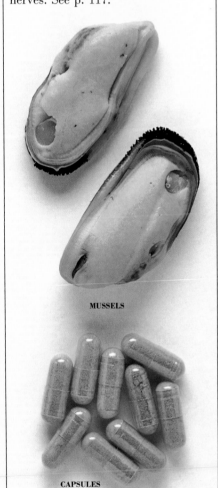

MUSSELS

CAPSULES

Perna canaliculata

GREEN-LIPPED MUSSEL

The sexual organs of the green-lipped mussel are a popular if unproven self-treatment for both rheumatoid and osteoarthritis. The mussels are taken as a powder in capsule form. See p. 117.

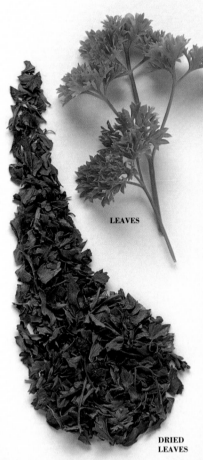

LEAVES

DRIED
LEAVES

Petroselinum crispum

PARSLEY

Valued by Culpeper for stomach, kidney, and menstrual problems, parsley leaves, roots, and seeds are still used by herbalists for urinary tract infections, kidney stones, poor digestion, and rheumatic complaints. See p. 118.

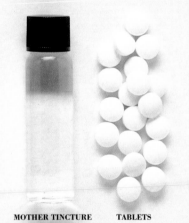

MOTHER TINCTURE   TABLETS

Phosphorus ☠

Homeopaths prescribe phosphorus – a nonmetallic, waxy mineral – for throat and lung disorders, including bronchitis and tonsillitis. They also use it for tinnitus (ringing noises in the ears), vomiting, and recurrent sties. See p. 118.

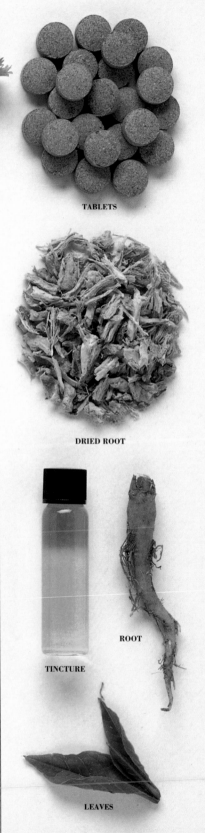

TABLETS

DRIED ROOT

TINCTURE

ROOT

LEAVES

Phytolacca decandra ☠

POKE ROOT

The dried root and berries are given by herbalists as tablets or a tincture for rheumatic and respiratory conditions. Homeopaths use *Phytolacca* for problems ranging from pain to dizziness. See p. 118.

PICRASMA EXCELSA

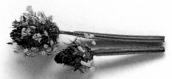

PLANTAIN FLOWER HEADS

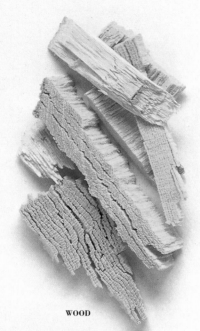

WOOD

Picrasma excelsa
JAMAICA QUASSIA
The wood of the Jamaica quassia tree is given by herbalists as a bitter (digestive stimulant) and a tonic when depressed health has caused poor appetite and digestion. Herbal medicine also uses it for treating parasitic infestations such as threadworms. See p. 118.

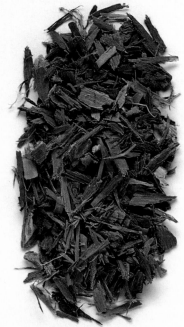

DRIED BARK

Piscidia piscipula
JAMAICAN DOGWOOD
The bark of this small Central American tree or shrub is used by herbalists for neuralgia, headache, menstrual cramps, and insomnia. It should be used only under the supervision of a qualified herbal practitioner. See p. 119.

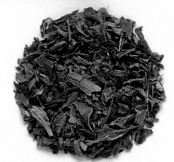

DRIED PLANTAIN LEAVES

ISPAGHULA SEEDS

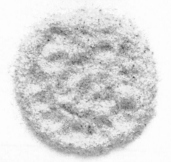

ISPAGHULA HUSKS

Plantago major & P. ovata
PLANTAIN; ISPAGHULA
Herbalists give plantain leaves for catarrh, cystitis, and hemorrhoids. Chinese physicians use plantain for urinary tract conditions. Ispaghula seeds are prescribed for chronic constipation and diarrhea in Indian and orthodox medicine. See p. 119.

DRIED CORAL

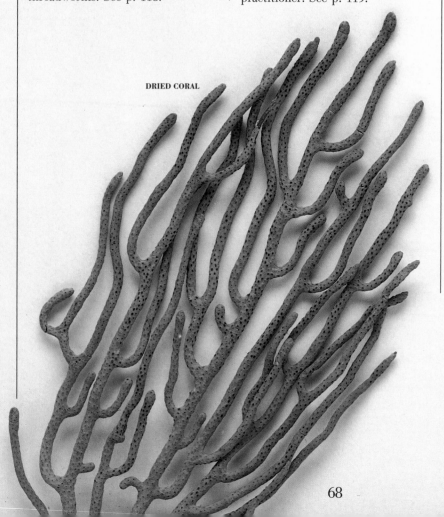

Plexaura species
SEA WHIP CORAL
The outer layers of sea whip coral contain prostaglandins, which are given to stimulate many body functions in orthodox medicine. Unani medicine values red coral for a wide range of illnesses, from palpitations and epilepsy to kidney stones and toothache. See p. 119.

PRUNUS SEROTINA

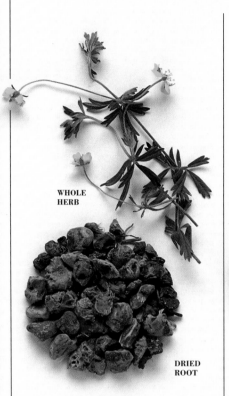

WHOLE HERB

DRIED ROOT

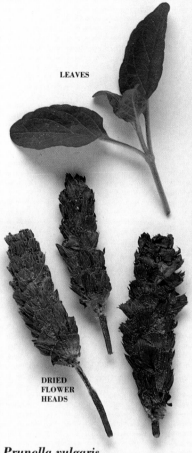

LEAVES

DRIED FLOWER HEADS

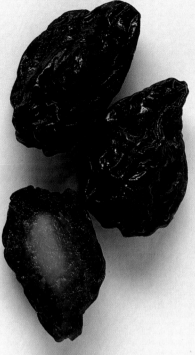

Potentilla erecta
TORMENTIL
This herb, used whole, is a long-established European remedy for colic, and is now given by herbalists as a treatment for diarrhea and stomach inflammation, as a mouthwash, and as a vaginal douche. See p. 119.

Prunella vulgaris
SELF HEAL
Self heal is both a name and a description for this long-used herb. It is still used by herbalists as a wound healer and to stop bleeding, and for conjunctivitis, high blood pressure, abscesses, and swelling in Chinese medicine. See p. 120.

Prunus domestica
PRUNE
Prunes are so widely used as a remedy for constipation that they are taken for granted. A perfect example of "let your food be your medicine," they are ideally suited as a gentle nutritive laxative for adults and children alike. See p. 120.

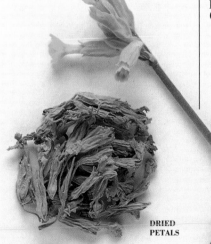

DRIED PETALS

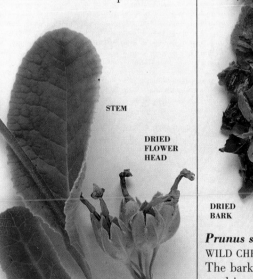

STEM

DRIED FLOWER HEAD

DRIED BARK

Primula veris
COWSLIP
The dried petals of cowslip, which flowers in early spring, have long been used medicinally in the herb's native northern Europe. Cowslip is given by herbalists for excitability, insomnia, bronchitis, and whooping cough. See p. 119.

Prunus serotina
WILD CHERRY
The bark of wild cherry has been used in cough syrups for centuries and is still employed by herbalists today for irritable and unproductive coughs. A related herb, *P. yedoensis*, is used for coughs in Chinese medicine. See p. 120.

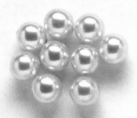

Pteria margaritifera
PEARL

Pearls – the result of an oyster's, clam's, or mussel's self-protection against an invader – are similar in composition to the lining of shell. As a powder, they are given by Chinese physicians for spasms, convulsions, headaches, and insomnia. See p. 120.

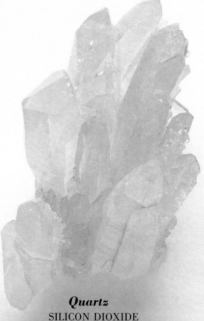

Quartz
SILICON DIOXIDE

Silicon dioxide is used as a non-active bulking agent in pharmaceutical tablets. Homeopaths use *Silicea* made from flint for a range of conditions, from debility due to overexertion to migraines. See p. 121.

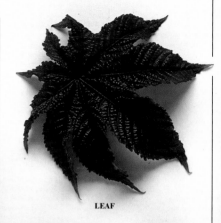

LEAF

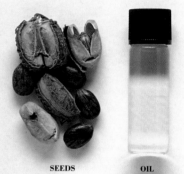

SEEDS   OIL

Ricinus communis ☠
CASTOR BEAN

The castor bean plant provided Victorians with castor oil to "clean out" the system. Herbalists still use the seeds for constipation, or in skin and eye lotions as a soother. Chinese physicians use the seeds, leaves, and root. See p. 121.

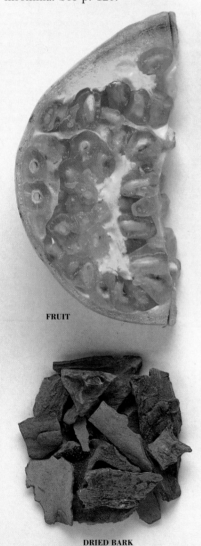

FRUIT

DRIED BARK

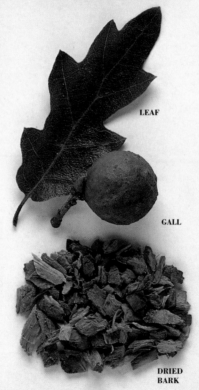

LEAF

GALL

DRIED BARK

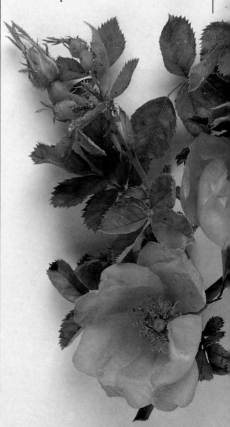

Punica granatum
POMEGRANATE

The rind of the pomegranate fruit, and the bark of its tree, are a pre-biblical remedy. They are prescribed by herbalists to treat intestinal worms and against amoebae. The bark is used against tapeworm and as a vaginal douche. See p. 120.

Quercus robur
ENGLISH OAK

The bark and galls of the English oak tree are given by herbalists for acute diarrhea, as a mouthwash for inflamed gums or ulcers, and as a vaginal douche, and applied locally on hemorrhoids, burns, and weeping wounds. See p. 121.

RUBUS IDAEUS

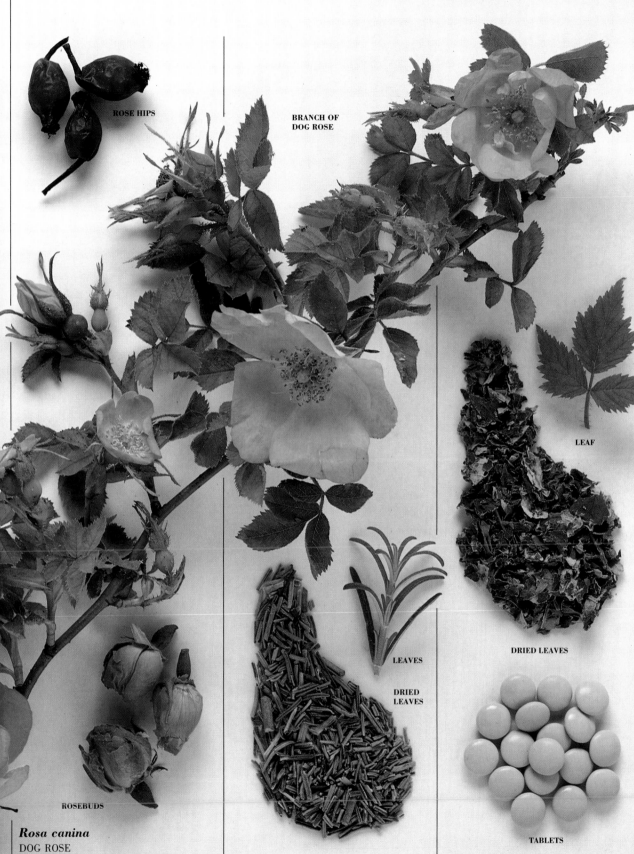

ROSE HIPS

BRANCH OF
DOG ROSE

LEAF

DRIED LEAVES

LEAVES

DRIED
LEAVES

ROSEBUDS

TABLETS

Rosa canina
DOG ROSE
The hips of the dog rose are one of the richest sources of vitamin C and are given by herbalists for colds and debility. They are also used herbally for mild diarrhea and stomach upsets. Rose petals from other *Rosa* species are used in rosewater to soothe the skin. See p. 121.

Rosmarinus officinalis
ROSEMARY
Long endowed with powers to influence life, rosemary is a key Mediterranean herb, whose leaves are used by herbalists for skin diseases, migraines, depression, and dandruff. See p. 121.

Rubus idaeus
RASPBERRY
Raspberry leaves, as a tea or tablets, can be taken during the last three months of pregnancy to ease childbirth. In Chinese medicine, they are used for diarrhea, pain, and amenorrhea. See p. 122.

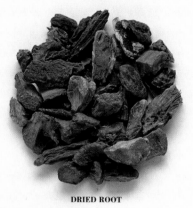

DRIED ROOT

Rumex crispus
YELLOW DOCK
The leaves and root of yellow dock
are given by herbalists as a gentle
laxative, and in chronic skin disease
linked with a sluggish liver or
bowel. Chinese medicine gives dock
for constipation, abdominal pain,
and cramps. See p. 122.

Saiga tatarica
ANTELOPE
Powder or pills of antelope horn
are given in Chinese medicine for
fevers, dizziness, blurred vision,
headaches, and convulsions.
Velvet from deer horn is
used as a tonic in Russian
medicine. See p. 122.

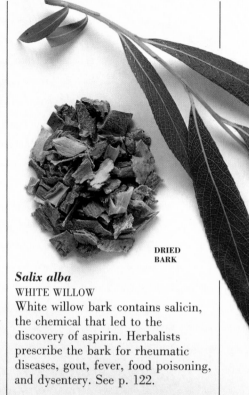

LEAVES

DRIED BARK

Salix alba
WHITE WILLOW
White willow bark contains salicin,
the chemical that led to the
discovery of aspirin. Herbalists
prescribe the bark for rheumatic
diseases, gout, fever, food poisoning,
and dysentery. See p. 122.

HORN

LEAF

DRIED LEAVES

Salvia officinalis
RED SAGE
A traditional cure-all, the leaves are
given by herbalists for a range of
conditions, from mouth and throat
infections to menopausal problems.
Chinese uses include insomnia,
hepatitis, and hives. See p. 122.

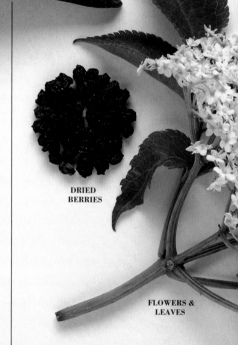

DRIED BERRIES

FLOWERS & LEAVES

Sambucus nigra
BLACK ELDER
The flowers, leaves, berries, and bark
of black elder all have herbal uses.
For example, the flowers relieve
symptoms of colds and flu. In
Chinese medicine, uses include leg
swelling and bone pain. See p. 123.

SCUTELLARIA LATERIFLORA

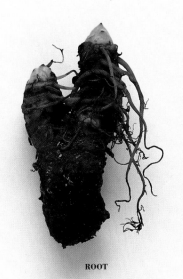

ROOT

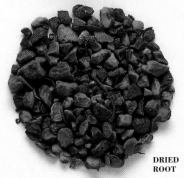

DRIED
ROOT

Sanguinaria canadensis ☠
BLOODROOT
The blood-colored root of this herb is given by herbalists for respiratory infections, and to remove benign skin tumors. Also, it is used in homeopathy for migraines. See p. 123.

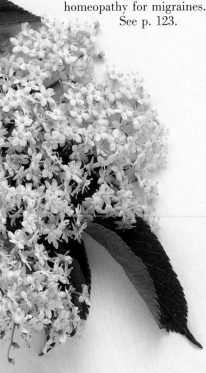

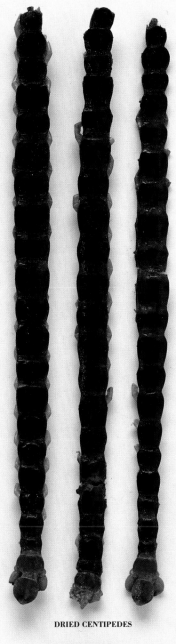

DRIED CENTIPEDES

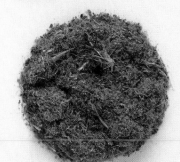

POWDERED CENTIPEDE

Scolopendra subspinipes mutilans
CENTIPEDE
Powdered whole centipede is used in Chinese prescriptions for convulsions, spasms, and lockjaw, and to counter poisoning. It is also applied externally for carbuncles, sores, and lumps. See p. 123.

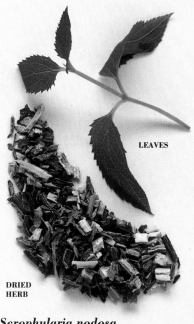

LEAVES

DRIED
HERB

Scrophularia nodosa
FIGWORT
Figwort got its botanical name from its traditional use as a treatment for scrofula (tuberculosis of the lymph glands). Herbalists now give the whole herb for poor circulation and chronic inflammatory conditions of the skin, such as eczema. See p. 123.

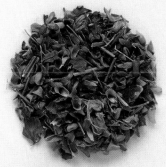

DRIED HERB

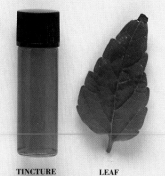

TINCTURE   LEAF

Scutellaria lateriflora
SKULLCAP
Called skullcap because of the bonnetlike shape of its dried calyx, the whole of this herb is given by herbalists for anxiety, nervous tension, and depression, and to reduce fits in epilepsy. See p. 124.

SELENIUM

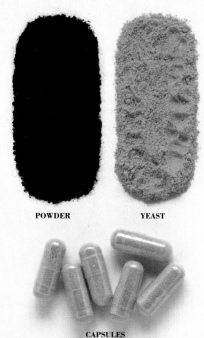

POWDER

YEAST

CAPSULES

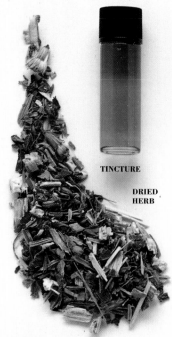

TINCTURE

DRIED HERB

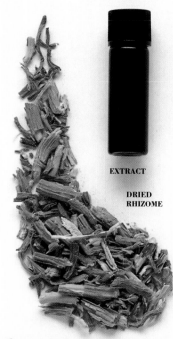

EXTRACT

DRIED RHIZOME

Selenium ☠

An essential trace element, selenium may make vitamin E more effective and is taken in capsule form as a supplement. Safe supplements are produced by growing yeast on selenium dioxide. Selenium sulfide is an active ingredient in dandruff shampoos. See p. 124.

Senecio aureus
LIFE ROOT

Used by Native Americans to treat vaginal discharges, life root is now also given by herbalists for menopausal problems and amenorrhea. The whole herb, including the small, yellow, daisylike flowers, is used. See p. 124.

Smilax species
SARSAPARILLA

Sarsaparilla root arrived in Europe in the 16th century as a treatment for syphilis. Herbalists now use it for chronic skin conditions such as psoriasis. Chinese medicine gives *S. glabra* and *S. china* for a variety of conditions. See p. 125.

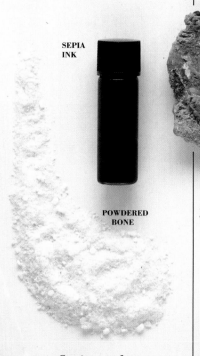

SEPIA INK

POWDERED BONE

BONE

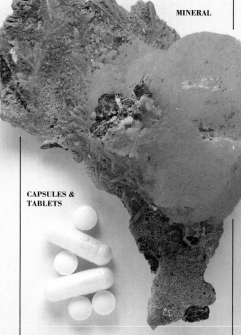

MINERAL

CAPSULES & TABLETS

Sepia esculenta
CUTTLEFISH

Cuttlefish bones are prescribed medicinally by Chinese and Unani physicians for a wide range of conditions. Sepia ink is used homeopathically. See p. 124.

Smithsonite
NATIVE ZINC CARBONATE

This natural form of zinc carbonate is a source for orthodox medicine's zinc supplements and zinc oxide cream for skin problems. In Chinese medicine, powdered smithsonite is used for skin problems. See p. 125.

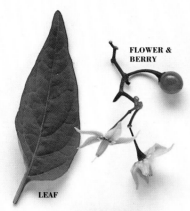

FLOWER & BERRY

LEAF

Solanum dulcamara ☠
BITTERSWEET
The stems of bittersweet, so named because its twigs taste bitter and then sweet, are a herbal remedy for rheumatism, psoriasis, eczema, and bronchitis. *Dulcamara* is given in homeopathy for conditions brought on by dampness or cold. See p. 125.

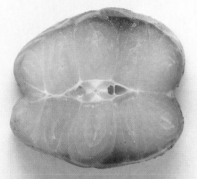

Somniosus microcephalus
GREENLAND SHARK-HORNED DOGFISH
Liver oil from this fish contains unusual fatty acids which trials have shown are valuable in reducing the side effects of cancer radiotherapy treatment. Chinese medicine uses it as a general tonic. See p. 125.

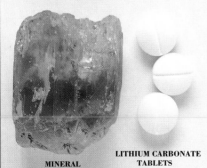

MINERAL

LITHIUM CARBONATE TABLETS

Spodumene
LITHIUM ALUMINUM SILICATE
Spodumene is a source of lithium, a nonessential mineral that is used in the form of lithium salts such as lithium carbonate to treat manic depression in orthodox medicine. See p. 125.

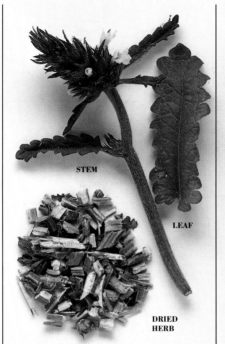

STEM

LEAF

DRIED HERB

Stachys betonica
BETONY
Betony, used medicinally since before the Romans, is given whole in herbal medicine for nervous headaches, digestive upsets in nervous states, and in liver and gallbladder disease. It is applied externally as a poultice to heal wounds and bruises. See p. 126.

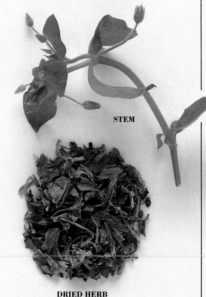

STEM

DRIED HERB

Stellaria media
CHICKWEED
Once used as a vegetable, chickweed is now applied externally as a herbal remedy for itchy and inflamed skin problems. The whole herb is also taken internally for rheumatic diseases. See p. 126.

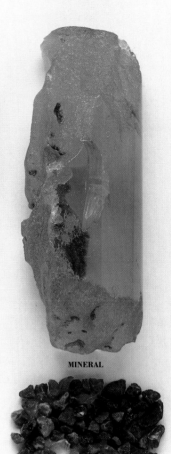

MINERAL

GROUND MINERAL

Succinum
AMBER
Amber, the fossilized gum of fir trees from some 300 million years ago, is given in Chinese medicine in ground form to treat conditions ranging from insomnia to urine retention. See p. 126.

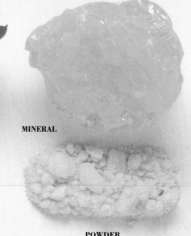

MINERAL

POWDER

Sulfur
As brimstone and treacle, sulfur has long been given as a laxative and "blood cleanser." It still has many uses in orthodox, Chinese, and homeopathic medicine, such as for skin problems and lack of stamina. See p. 126.

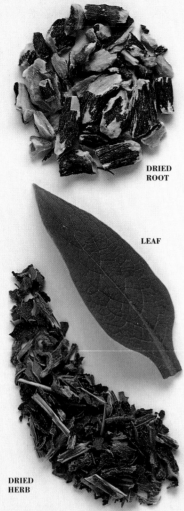

DRIED
ROOT

LEAF

DRIED
HERB

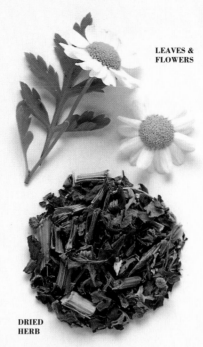

LEAVES &
FLOWERS

DRIED
HERB

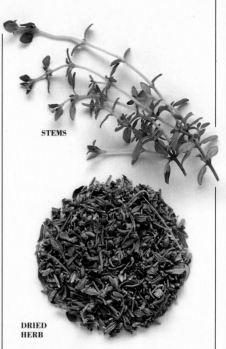

STEMS

DRIED
HERB

Symphytum officinale
COMFREY
One of the best-established herbal remedies for the treatment of wounds, sprains, and strains, it is also used to heal broken bones, hence its other common name, knitbone. See p. 127.

Tanacetum parthenium
FEVERFEW
The whole herb has recently been rediscovered as a preventive treatment for migraines. It is also given in herbal medicine for arthritis, menstrual cramps, and after childbirth to help restore the uterus. See p. 127.

Thymus species
THYME
Flowering thyme is one of the oldest herbal remedies; it is given for coughs, bronchitis, and indigestion. A natural antiseptic, it is also used as a gargle for throat infections and as an infusion to disinfect wounds. See p. 128.

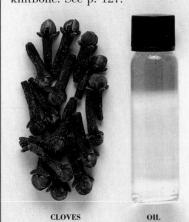

CLOVES

OIL

Syzigium aromaticum
CLOVES
Cloves, the dried buds of this evergreen tree, contain an oil which is widely used to relieve toothache. Herbalists also give it internally for digestive problems. See p. 127.

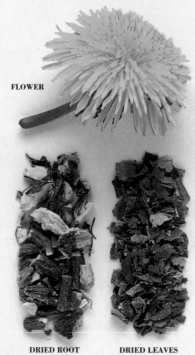

FLOWER

DRIED ROOT

DRIED LEAVES

Taraxacum officinalis
DANDELION
Dandelion root and leaves provide one of the safest and most effective herbal diuretics. They are also used for many other conditions in herbal and Chinese medicine. See p. 127.

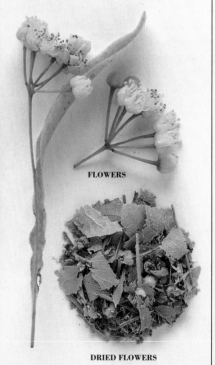

FLOWERS

DRIED FLOWERS

Tilia x europea
SMALL-LEAVED EUROPEAN LINDEN
Linden flower tea is widely used in Europe as a relaxing drink. Herbalists also give it for fevers, colds, and flu. It is especially useful for children. See p. 128.

TUSSILAGO FARFARA

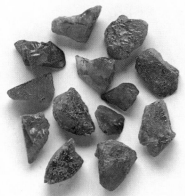

Titanite
CALCIUM TITANIUM SILICATE
This mineral is a main source of titanium, which is used to make titanium dioxide, an important ingredient in suntan products. Titanium can absorb ultraviolet light, shielding the skin and preventing sunburn. See p. 128.

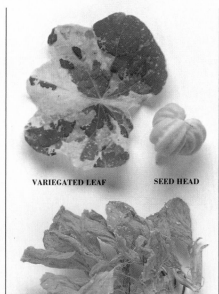

VARIEGATED LEAF   SEED HEAD

DRIED FLOWERS

Tropaeolum majus
NASTURTIUM
Nasturtium seeds were brought to Europe from Peru in the 16th century. The whole herb or fresh leaves are used by herbalists for infections of the urinary tract and the respiratory system, and as an antiseptic. See p. 128.

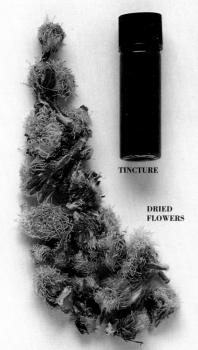

TINCTURE

DRIED FLOWERS

Tussilago farfara
COLTSFOOT
The leaves and flowers have provided herbalists with a cough remedy since the ancient Greeks — *tussis* means cough in Greek. They are still given by herbalists to soothe dry, irritable coughs, asthma, and bronchitis. See p. 129.

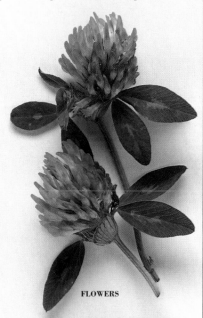

FLOWERS

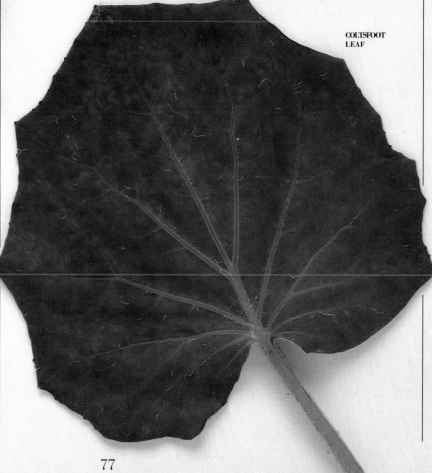

COLTSFOOT LEAF

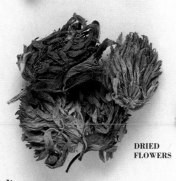

DRIED FLOWERS

Trifolium pratense
RED CLOVER
The flowers of red clover were first used medicinally by Native Americans, even though the plant is native to Europe. Herbally, it is used for skin diseases, including psoriasis and eczema. See p. 128.

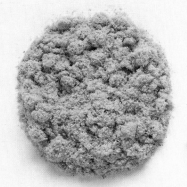

POWDER

Ulmus rubra
SLIPPERY ELM

The inner bark of slippery elm, originally used by Native Americans, is given internally by herbalists to soothe sore throats or an irritated digestive tract. It is also applied to boils and infected wounds as a poultice. See p. 129.

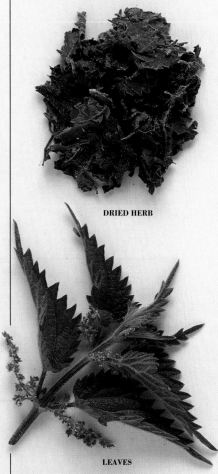

DRIED HERB

LEAVES

Urtica dioica
STINGING NETTLE

The common nettle is used by herbalists to treat skin disease and rheumatism. The sting is deactivated by drying or heating. Homeopaths give *U. urens* for rheumatism, burns, and rashes. See p. 129.

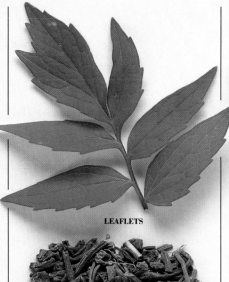

LEAFLETS

DRIED ROOT

Valeriana officinalis
VALERIAN

Valerian root is one of the most well-known herbal treatments for all kinds of nervous conditions, such as anxiety. Chinese physicians also give it for traumatic injury, flu, and rheumatism. See p. 129.

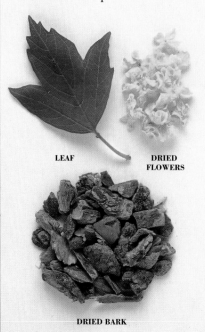

LEAF DRIED FLOWERS

DRIED BARK

Viburnum opulus
CRAMP BARK

The bark of beautiful white-flowered cramp bark, or guelder rose, has long been given by herbalists for menstrual and general cramping. American *V. prunifolium* is used in the same way. See p. 130.

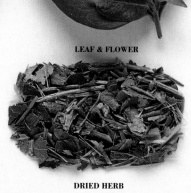

LEAF & FLOWER

DRIED HERB

Vinca major
GREATER PERIWINKLE

The whole herb is given internally by herbalists to treat excessive menstrual bleeding and externally for hemorrhoids and nosebleeds. Related *V. minor* is given homeopathically. See p. 130.

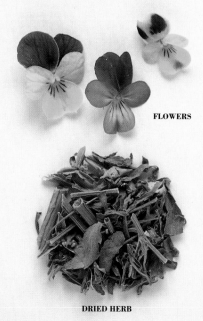

FLOWERS

DRIED HERB

Viola tricolor
HEARTSEASE

This herb is an example of how shape can lead to usage; the heart-shaped flowers were traditionally used to mend broken hearts. Its herbal uses now include bronchitis, rheumatism, and gout. See p. 130.

ZINGIBER OFFICINALIS

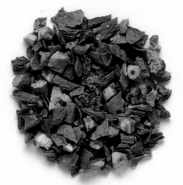

DRIED LEAVES

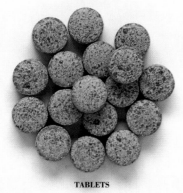

TABLETS

DRIED BARK

TABLETS

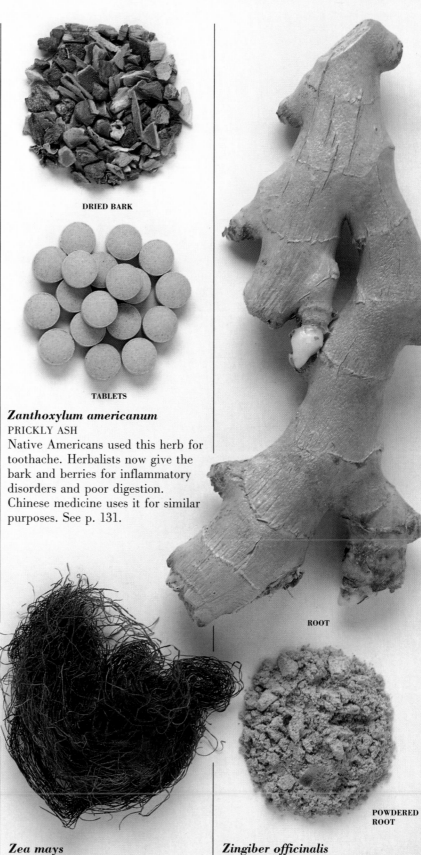

ROOT

Viscum album
MISTLETOE
The leaves and berries of mistletoe are dried and given as tablets, a decoction, or a tincture for high blood pressure linked with arterial disease, especially when nervous conditions are present. See p. 130.

Zanthoxylum americanum
PRICKLY ASH
Native Americans used this herb for toothache. Herbalists now give the bark and berries for inflammatory disorders and poor digestion. Chinese medicine uses it for similar purposes. See p. 131.

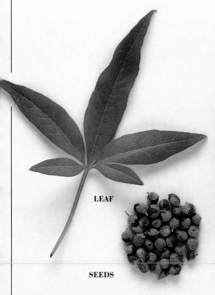

LEAF

SEEDS

POWDERED ROOT

Vitex agnus-castus
CHASTEBERRY
The seeds of this Mediterranean shrub are given by herbalists to help balance the female hormonal system, whether the problem concerns the menstrual cycle or menopause. The plant is also reputed to reduce the sex urge in men. See p. 131.

Zea mays
CORN
Corn silk from the maize plant is a key herbal remedy for inflammatory conditions of the urinary tract, such as cystitis, bladder, and kidney infections, and kidney stones. See p. 131.

Zingiber officinalis
GINGER
Ginger root, used medicinally since the ancient Greeks, is a worldwide herbal remedy. It is given for poor peripheral (local) circulation, lung infections, indigestion, flatulence, and motion sickness. See p. 131.

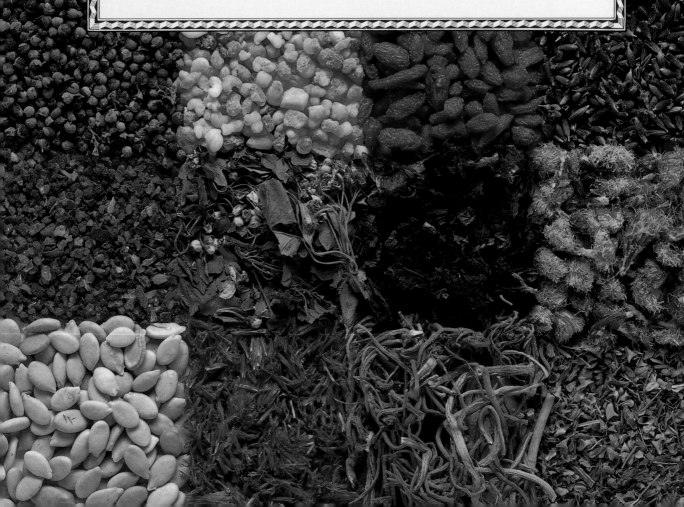

Reference Guide to the A–Z

A systematic listing of all the ingredients featured in the A–Z, with information on their characteristics, properties, and the symptoms and disorders they are used to treat.

How to Use This Section

The Reference Guide provides detailed profiles of all the animals, minerals, and plants illustrated in the A–Z of Nature's Medicine Chest, which were chosen to reflect the enormous diversity of healing ingredients and the range of illnesses and symptoms for which they are given. Their selection was based on two main criteria: that they are currently in use in at least one of the main healing systems, these being herbal medicine, Chinese herbalism, Indian medicine, homeopathy, and orthodox medicine; and that there is evidence of their healing value, whether from a long history of empirical observation or from recent experimental analysis. Each entry is presented under the headings explained below. Unfamiliar terms, if not explained here, can be found in the glossary on pp. 138–9.

Sample entry

Latin name
Each entry is ordered by its Latin name. This is an internationally accepted language of identification. Latin names separated by "/" are synonyms, and those separated by "&" are different species within the same family. When repeated, the species name is shortened to the first letter. The family name is given in brackets.

Common names
The most widely used common names are given, some reflecting the medical uses of the material.

Parts used
Only rarely is the entire plant or animal used; usually particular parts contain all or most of the medically useful substances, which are listed. Unless otherwise stated, the part used is fresh.

Medicinal use
The main professional use of each remedy. The uses given are those of herbal medicine unless otherwise stated. When a remedy is used homeopathically, the name is given in italics in brackets.

Symbol
Indicates whether the remedy is a plant (✦), mineral (◉), or animal (✺) and, in some cases, whether it is a poison (☠).

Introduction
A profile of the ingredient's origin, historical uses, and a thumbnail description where appropriate.

Active ingredients
While the chemical content of minerals is easily analyzed, the same is not true of plants and animals, which contain thousands of chemical compounds. This section lists those substances known to be in the remedy and thought to be involved in its healing effects.

Actions
The known healing actions of the active ingredients.

Preparations
The common forms in which active ingredients are extracted efficiently and made available in a way that is effective and convenient to use.

Caution
All medicines should be treated with respect. Entries that must be used with particular care are identified with a caution and should not be used without professional advice.

Aconitum napellus (Ranunculaceae) ✦☠

ACONITE, MONKSHOOD, WOLF'S BANE

The ancient Chinese used this deadly herb as an arrow poison, and the name aconite is thought to have come from the Latin for dart. A native of central and southern Europe, it is an attractive garden perennial with dark green, deeply divided leaves and deep blue-purple flowers on a spike.

PARTS USED: Dried root, collected in the autumn.

ACTIVE INGREDIENTS: Alkaloids, including aconitine and traces of ephedrine.

ACTIONS: Sedative; relieves pain.

MEDICINAL USE: Poisonous to the heart and nervous system, it is rarely used internally except in homeopathic doses (*Aconite*) at the start of acute illnesses such as flu, colds, or measles, and in emergencies. It is applied externally to relieve the pain of bruising, sciatica, rheumatism, and neuralgia, but should never be applied to broken skin. Chinese medicine uses a tincture of several species of *Aconitum* as a local anesthetic and prescribes it internally for heart disease, but with the poisonous aconitine removed.

PREPARATIONS: Tincture, lotion, homeopathic remedies.

CAUTION: **Highly poisonous; U.S. law prohibits its sale and professional use. Medicinal use in Canada is not legal.**

Achillea millefolium (Compositae)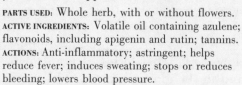
YARROW, MILFOIL, NOSEBLEED,
STAUNCH WEED

The Latin name for yarrow is said to have
arisen because Achilles used the herb to stop
his soldiers' wounds from bleeding. Native
to Europe, yarrow has spread to many
temperate regions, and, like most weeds,
grows readily on any waste ground. The
stem is angular with a profusion of long
green-gray leaves that look like fern fronds.
Small white or pink-tinged flowers with
yellow centers appear in summer.

PARTS USED: Whole herb, with or without flowers.
ACTIVE INGREDIENTS: Volatile oil containing azulene;
flavonoids, including apigenin and rutin; tannins.
ACTIONS: Anti-inflammatory; astringent; helps
reduce fever; induces sweating; stops or reduces
bleeding; lowers blood pressure.
MEDICINAL USE: Given to help the body control
fevers, flu, and the common cold. Also used for
high blood pressure, stomach ulcers, amenorrhea,
and as a poultice for minor cuts and abrasions.
PREPARATIONS: Infusion, tincture, poultice.

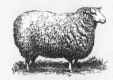

Adeps lanae

Aconitum napellus (Ranunculaceae)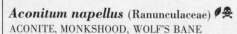
ACONITE, MONKSHOOD, WOLF'S BANE

The ancient Chinese used this deadly herb
as an arrow poison, and the name aconite is
thought to have come from the Latin for
dart. A native of central and southern
Europe, it is an attractive garden perennial
with dark green, deeply divided leaves and
deep blue-purple flowers on a spike.

PARTS USED: Dried root, collected in the autumn.
ACTIVE INGREDIENTS: Alkaloids, including aconitine
and traces of ephedrine.
ACTIONS: Sedative; relieves pain.
MEDICINAL USE: Poisonous to the heart and nervous
system, it is rarely used internally except in
homeopathic doses (*Aconite*) at the start of acute
illnesses like flu, and in emergencies. It is applied
externally to relieve the pain of bruising, sciatica,
rheumatism, and neuralgia, but should never be
applied to broken skin. Chinese medicine uses a
tincture of several species of *Aconitum* as a local
anesthetic and prescribes it internally for heart
disease, but with poisonous aconitine removed.
PREPARATIONS: Tincture, lotion, homeopathic
remedies.
CAUTION: **Highly poisonous; U.S. law prohibits
its sale and professional use. Medicinal use in
Canada is not legal.**

Actinolite
A handsome green, actinolite crystals are
common throughout the world. They can be
opaque, translucent, or glassy.

PARTS USED: Crystals.
ACTIVE INGREDIENTS: Complex silicate of calcium,
magnesium, and iron.
ACTIONS: Tonic; reduces muscle tension and
spasms.
MEDICINAL USE: Chinese medicine prescribes
actinolite for colic, muscle cramps, prostatitis

(inflammation of the prostate gland),
endometritis (inflammation of the uterine lining),
amenorrhea, and impotence.
PREPARATIONS: Powder, pills, decoction.

Adeps lanae
WOOL FAT, ANHYDROUS LANOLIN

Many cosmetics, soaps, leather preparations,
and medicines contain lanolin, the waxy
coating that makes sheep's wool waterproof
and warm. However, in spite of its
usefulness, lanolin is one of the most
common allergy-causing substances and is
therefore usually labelled on skin
preparations. Raw wool contains
considerable quantities of crude lanolin,
which is boiled off and refined.

PARTS USED: Wool fat.
ACTIVE INGREDIENTS: Cholesterol; monohydric
alcohols; cetyl, ceryl, and carnaubyl alcohols.
ACTIONS: Softens and soothes the skin.
MEDICINAL USE: Used as an emollient base for
medicated creams and ointments, to soften and
soothe the skin, and to improve the absorption of
a drug through the skin.
PREPARATIONS: Ointment, liquid.

Agathosma betulina/Barosma betulina
(Rutaceae)
BUCHU LEAVES

A. betulina is a small shrub native to Cape
Province in South Africa, where the local
Hottentots use its leaves mixed with oil as a
body perfume. The pale green leaves are
rounded with a curved point and have a
leathery feel; oil glands can be seen on their
surface. The flowers are small and white,
but are rarely seen in samples of the herb.

PARTS USED: Dried leaves, collected during
flowering.
ACTIVE INGREDIENTS: Volatile oil containing
diosphenol, pulegone, and limonene; flavonoids
such as rutin, hesperidin, and quercitin; tannins.
ACTIONS: Increases urine production; urinary
antiseptic.
MEDICINAL USE: Given for cystitis, other
inflammatory conditions of the urinary tract, and
for prostatitis (inflammation of the prostate
gland). However, it should not be used when
there is kidney infection.
PREPARATIONS: Infusion, tincture.

Agkistrodon rhodostoma &
A. acutus
PIT VIPER

The snake's long use in medicine is marked
by its presence in many modern symbols of
medicine – a snake entwining a staff, taken
from Hippocrates. Pit vipers are the snakes
employed most often in medicine; at least
five species are used. *A. acutus*, native to
southeast China, Vietnam, and Taiwan, and
A. rhodostoma, the Malayan pit viper, are
renowned for their dangerous venom.

PARTS USED: Venom, oil, cooked flesh of headless body, whole body.

ACTIVE INGREDIENTS: Enzymes; ancrod.

ACTIONS: Tonic; reduces muscle tension and spasms; relieves pain; prevents blood clotting.

MEDICINAL USE: The main use of venom is to extract antivenin to treat snake bites, from which 30,000 people die each year. In Unani medicine, viper flesh is given to strengthen eyesight, ease muscular pains, and improve intelligence, and the venom is prescribed as a slow-acting but long-lasting painkiller to relieve chronic pain such as sciatica. Chinese medicine favors local *A. acutus* to treat spasms, tremors, seizures, joint stiffness and weakness, cramps, and facial paralysis. Ancrod is extracted pharmaceutically from enzymes in *A. rhodostoma* venom and given in orthodox medicine to discourage the formation of blood clots that may cause stroke or heart attack.

PREPARATIONS: *Unani:* cooked flesh of headless body, or a paste of snake ash with honey for eyesight. *Chinese:* powdered dried snake. *Orthodox:* injection.

Agrimonia eupatoria (Rosaceae)
AGRIMONY, COCKLEBUR, STICKLEWORT

Agrimony has been a popular medicinal herb throughout history; one ancient recipe suggested mixing it with human blood and frogs to stop internal bleeding. Its leaves, which the French value as a tisane, have a delicate aroma. Agrimony grows wild all over Europe, Asia, and North America, especially on dry waste ground. It has attractive hairy, divided leaves at ground level and a tall spike with bright yellow flowers in the summer. The flowers produce fruit covered in tough hairs, which stick to passing animals or clothes.

PARTS USED: Stems, leaves.

ACTIVE INGREDIENTS: Tannins; coumarins; volatile oil; flavonoids, including apigenin and quercitin.

ACTIONS: Astringent; increases urine production.

MEDICINAL USE: Used against diarrhea in children and mucous colitis (an inflammatory condition of the intestines), as a poultice for ulcers and slowly healing wounds, and as a gargle in acute sore throats. Given for tuberculosis and internal bleeding by Chinese physicians.

PREPARATIONS: Infusion, tincture, gargle, poultice.

Agropyron repens (Graminae)
WITCHGRASS, COUCHGRASS, QUACK GRASS

A notorious garden weed throughout the world, it is native to Europe but traveled with early explorers and settlers. The roots have been used as a medicine since Dioscorides in 77 AD, and even sick dogs eat the leaves to produce a healing vomit. In Europe, it is still used as a tisane. Long white rhizomes spread as a dense mat in the soil and produce clumps of grass blades. In midsummer, a flowering spike appears with two rows of closely packed small flowers that look like rye.

PARTS USED: Rhizome, collected in the spring.

ACTIVE INGREDIENTS: A polysaccharide, triticin, and other carbohydrates such as inositol, mannitol, and mucilage; volatile oil containing agropyrene.

ACTIONS: Soothing; increases urine production.

MEDICINAL USE: Used for painful urinary tract problems, including inflammatory urinary tract conditions such as cystitis, kidney stones, and prostatitis (inflammation of the prostate gland).

PREPARATIONS: Decoction, tincture.

Alchemilla vulgaris (Rosaceae)
LADY'S MANTLE

The Latin name for lady's mantle comes from the Arabic for alchemy, which hints at the medicinal value of the herb. Native to Britain, it is widely distributed across northern Europe. The plant is perennial, covered in soft hairs, and has beautiful lobed, kidney-shaped leaves. From early to midsummer, tiny yellow-green flowers appear in clusters on long stalks.

PARTS USED: Leaves, flowering tops.

ACTIVE INGREDIENTS: Tannins.

ACTIONS: Astringent; stops bleeding from external wounds.

MEDICINAL USE: Given internally for diarrhea and heavy menstruation. It is applied as a douche for leukorrhea (excessive, pale white vaginal discharge) and vaginal pruritis (itching), and used as a mouthwash for bleeding gums, and as a gargle for laryngitis.

PREPARATIONS: Infusion for douche, mouthwash, gargle, tincture.

Allium sativum (Liliaceae)
GARLIC

Garlic has been a culinary and medicinal herb for so long that its origins have been lost in time. The pharaohs are said to have had it placed in their own tombs and also to have fed it to their slaves for strength. The ancient Greeks and Romans used it as medicine, and Culpeper described it as "a remedy for all diseases and hurts." Medical journals regularly publish scientific studies confirming the medicinal properties of garlic. It is native to Siberia, and to southern Europe where it is almost a staple food. The leaves are flat and thin, and a spherical flower head of tiny greenish white or pink flowers appears in midsummer. The bulb is covered in white papery skin and comprises 8 to 15 segments, or cloves.

PARTS USED: Cloves.

ACTIVE INGREDIENTS: Volatile oil containing sulfur compounds, particularly alliin, which converts to allicin and then aloen when a clove is crushed; geraniol and linalool.

ACTIONS: Antiseptic; antibacterial; expectorant; antiviral; induces sweating; kills and helps expel worms; lowers blood pressure and cholesterol levels; reduces blood clotting in blood vessels.

MEDICINAL USE: Used for coughs, colds, bronchitis, and catarrh; regular use may help prevent colds

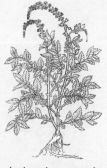

Agrimonia eupatoria

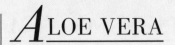

by strengthening the immune system. Garlic is also given to help control blood pressure and blood cholesterol levels. Prescribed in Chinese medicine for tuberculosis, coughs, and digestive complaints such as diarrhea.
PREPARATIONS: Fresh cloves, tablets of powdered garlic, capsules of oil, tincture, syrup.

Aloe vera/A. barbadensis (Liliaceae) ✿
ALOE

Recent cosmetic fashion for aloe creams and shampoos belies the herb's ancient history; Aristotle had Alexander the Great studying how the Socotra islanders extracted aloe juice as long ago as 325 BC. There are over 200 varieties of aloe used, most deriving from species native to East and West Africa. A succulent perennial, the plant has whorls of thick fleshy leaves, usually with a toothed margin, often without a stem, and filled with bitter juice. A flower spike, growing 2 to 3 feet tall and terminating in an elongated cluster of trumpet-shaped, yellow or red flowers, appears in the summer.

PARTS USED: Juice and mucilage from the leaves.
ACTIVE INGREDIENTS: Anthraquinone glycosides (known as aloin), including aloe-emodin, aloin A and B, and aloinside; sterols; saponins; resin.
ACTIONS: Juice purges the bowels; mucilage softens and soothes the skin, and promotes wound healing.
MEDICINAL USE: The fresh mucilage is applied directly to burns, slow-healing wounds, and inflamed skin. Aloe's purgative action is so strong that the herb is rarely used internally alone, but is usually given with antispasmodics such as *Atropa belladonna* (p. 88) to stop colic. Chinese medicine prescribes it as a laxative and to stimulate the stomach.
PREPARATIONS: Powder, tablets, cream, fresh juice.

Althaea officinalis (Malvaceae) ✿
MARSH MALLOW, MORTIFICATION ROOT

An ancient food plant as well as a medicine, marsh mallow is mentioned in the Bible and in Arabic and Chinese history as a valuable food for the poor and in famines. The ancient Greeks used it as both a medicine and a decoration for graves, and it is widely used in European folk medicine. A perennial shrub, it has a thick, white, tapering root, pale green, lobed leaves, and pale pink, five-petalled flowers in late summer. Unlike other common mallow species, its leaves and stems are covered in soft down.

PARTS USED: Roots collected in autumn from two-year-old plants; leaves.
ACTIVE INGREDIENTS: Polysaccharide mucilage; pectin; flavonoids (in leaves), quercitin, and kaempferol; phenolic acids such as salicylic acid.
ACTIONS: Soothes internal body surfaces; softens and soothes the skin; expectorant; promotes wound healing.
MEDICINAL USE: Given internally for catarrh, bronchitis, irritating cough, gastritis (stomach

inflammation), peptic ulcers, and in urinary tract infections and irritations such as cystitis. Applied externally as a poultice for boils, carbuncles, and varicose ulcers.
PREPARATIONS: Infusion, decoction, tincture, poultice.

Aluminum, potassium, & sodium silicates 🔷
PUMICE

This extraordinary light volcanic lava results from stone being heated until it is soft. Then, as it cools, the stone becomes spongy as steam escapes. Pumice stones are widely used cosmetically to remove dead skin and are also used in dentistry.

PARTS USED: Whole pumice.
ACTIVE INGREDIENTS: Aluminum, potassium, and sodium silicates.
ACTIONS: Sedative; expectorant; drives phlegm from lungs; cooling; abrasive.
MEDICINAL USE: In Chinese medicine, it is given for any ailment that produces phlegm or sputum, such as bronchitis, and to encourage urination.
PREPARATIONS: Powder.

Amanita muscaria (Agariaceae) ✿☠
FLY AGARIC

One of the most ancient hallucinogens, fly agaric was used by the Siberian shamans (medicine men) to induce ecstatic and visionary states. The Lapps take it regularly and discovered that its active chemicals pass unchanged in the urine, which can be drunk for repeated effects. The common name comes from the use of its toxic contents to kill flies and other insects. Easily recognized by its bright red cap with white flecking, fly agaric has white gills and a white stem. Like many fungi, it grows in temperate woodlands, especially in autumn.

PARTS USED: Fresh fungus or dried cap.
ACTIVE INGREDIENTS: Muscarine; muscimol; ibotenic acid.
ACTIONS: Affects the central nervous system, causing twitching, vomiting, comatose states, and hallucinations.
MEDICINAL USE: Used only in homeopathic doses (*Agaricus muscarius*) for neurological problems characterized by involuntary movements.
PREPARATIONS: Homeopathic remedies.
CAUTION: **Highly toxic, handle with care.**

Anacardium occidentale (Anacardiaceae) ✿
CASHEW NUT

As with many tropical forest trees, different parts of the cashew tree are used locally for a range of purposes, from insecticide to ink, as well as in medicine. Native to South American jungles, the cashew is cultivated in the tropical zones of other countries. The tree grows to 40 feet and has blunt oval leaves. When its small, yellowish pink

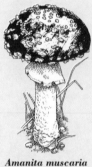

Amanita muscaria

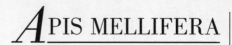

flowers fall, their receptacles swell and produce a kidney-shaped grayish fruit containing the cashew nut kernel.

PARTS USED: Bark, juice, and oil from fruit, kernels.
ACTIVE INGREDIENTS: Protein; niacin; anacardic acid; cardol; magnesium; iron.
ACTIONS: Bark extracts help to reduce fever; oil from the fruit dissolves protein in dead skin; fruit juice increases urine production; kernels are nutritive.
MEDICINAL USE: The oil can be used to remove warts, corns, ringworm, and cancerous ulcers. The fruit juice has been used in uterine complaints. It is also given in homeopathic doses (*Anacardium*) for anxiety, breathing difficulties, and digestive tract disorders.
PREPARATIONS: Fresh juice, oil, dried kernels, decoction of bark, homeopathic remedies.
CAUTION: **The oil is corrosive, use with care.**

Anemone pulsatilla/Pulsatilla vulgaris (Ranunculaceae) 🌢☠

PASQUEFLOWER, WINDFLOWER, MEADOW ANEMONE, PRAIRIE ANEMONE, WILD CROCUS

Named after its habit of flowering at Easter, the pasqueflower has been used in medicine since at least the time of the ancient Greeks. It is native to northern Europe and thrives on chalky soils. A perennial, it has leathery leaves growing in a rosette and covered in long hairs, a thick root, and purple flowers.

PARTS USED: Dried whole herb.
ACTIVE INGREDIENTS: Glycoside (ranunculin in fresh herb, which converts to anemonin on drying); saponins; tannins; resin.
ACTIONS: Sedative; relieves pain; reduces muscle tension and spasms; kills bacteria.
MEDICINAL USE: Given to relieve tense and painful conditions of the male and female reproductive systems, such as menstrual cramps, orchitis (inflammation of the testicles), and prostatitis (inflammation of the prostate gland). Also used for tension headache, hyperactivity, insomnia, and earache. Used in homeopathy (*Pulsatilla*) for catarrh, indigestion, measles, and for conditions characterized by weepiness and indecision, and by Chinese physicians for diarrhea.
PREPARATIONS: Infusion, decoction, tincture, tablets, homeopathic remedies.
CAUTION: **Fresh is poisonous, use only dried.**

Angelica archangelica (Umbelliferae) 🌢
ANGELICA

The crystallized stems of angelica are used in candy making and in liqueurs such as Chartreuse and vermouth. Its medicinal use was not popular until the 15th century, when it was used mainly against the "plague and all epidemical diseases." It was seen as a wonder plant and Culpeper recommended it for conditions ranging from dog bites to gout. Native to northern Europe, it is biennial, with a thick, fleshy root, hollow stems, toothed leaves, and clusters of greenish flowers in late summer.

PARTS USED: Dried root and seeds, fresh leaves and stems.
ACTIVE INGREDIENTS: Volatile oils containing pinene and cymene; valerianic acid; coumarins; iridoids; resin; tannins.
ACTIONS: Reduces muscle tension and spasms; induces sweating; expectorant; bitter (digestive stimulant); relieves gas and colic; increases urine production.
MEDICINAL USE: Given for catarrh, bronchitis, flatulence, and indigestion, and also used as a digestive and liver tonic. Several related species are prescribed in Chinese medicine for colds, headaches, arthritis, and rheumatism, and in Ayurvedic medicine for digestive problems and circulatory conditions.
PREPARATIONS: Infusion, tincture.

Aphanes arvensis (Rosaceae) 🌢
PARSLEY PIERT, BREAKSTONE

The common name breakstone comes from the herb's centuries-old use to break down kidney stones. Native to Britain, it is common throughout northern Europe, where it grows on dry, barren ground. It is a prostrate annual with clusters of three-lobed, green leaves and insignificant green flowers that appear in the summer.

PARTS USED: Whole herb, collected during flowering.
ACTIVE INGREDIENTS: Astringent principle, probably mainly tannins.
ACTIONS: Increases urine production; soothes internal body surfaces; breaks up kidney stones.
MEDICINAL USE: Used to dissolve kidney or bladder stones and to soothe a urinary tract irritated by the presence or the passage of stones.
PREPARATIONS: Infusion, tincture.

Apis mellifera ⚥
HONEYBEE

The honeybee has always been recognized by man as one of his most valuable allies. By far its greatest contributions are the pollination of crops, followed by the provision of several intriguing substances that help human health.

PARTS USED: Bee venom and venom extract; whole body; honey; beeswax; propolis, the sticky resin collected by bees from plants to glue up holes in the hive; royal jelly, a bitter-tasting gel secreted to feed infant queen bees; bee pollen.
ACTIVE INGREDIENTS: Melittin in venom and whole body; inhibine in honey; beeswax; propolis; pantothenic acid (B vitamin) and acetylcholine in royal jelly; bee pollen.
ACTIONS: Counterirritant (melittin, whole body); antibiotic (melittin, inhibine, propolis, royal jelly); tonic (whole body, royal jelly, bee pollen); laxative (honey); soothes internal body surfaces (honey); sedative (honey); anti-inflammatory (beeswax); stimulates the stomach (beeswax); relieves pain (beeswax); neutralizes toxic substances (beeswax).
MEDICINAL USE: Venom has been used traditionally for arthritis, and venom extract is prescribed as an antidote for bee stings in people dangerously

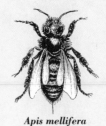

Apis mellifera

allergic to them. Wingless dried bee is given in Unani medicine as a tonic or applied externally on stings and skin inflammation. Whole bee (*Apis mel*) is used homeopathically for painful inflammatory conditions and swellings. Honey is universally valued for wound, external ulcer, and burn healing, is associated with longevity and vitality, is given for constipation where a gentle action is important, and is used for coughs and bronchitis. Beeswax is given by Chinese and Unani physicians for similar purposes. In the West, herbalists prescribe wax cappings, taken from the surface of honeycombs and containing some pollen, for hay-fever sufferers to build up their immunity. Propolis dates back at least to the time of Aristotle as an application for bruises, wounds, skin inflammation, and burns. It is now taken for mouth and stomach ulcers. Royal jelly has been associated with hormonal effects, but these are unproven; its best-established effect is as a general tonic. Bee pollen is taken for a range of problems, from impotence to depression, but its most general use is to build up the body's immunity to pollen.

PREPARATIONS: *Whole bees:* bee stings from live bees. *Venom/melittin:* injections. *Honey:* with or without wax comb (honey in jars, which has been heated to enable debris to be filtered out, may have lost useful enzymes and other volatile ingredients). *Wax cappings:* in jars. *Beeswax:* raw or in hand and face creams. *Propolis:* tablets, lozenges, liquid extract. *Royal jelly:* tablets, ampules of fresh chilled jelly. *Bee pollen:* grains, tablets.

Arctium lappa (Compositae)
GREAT BURDOCK, BEGGAR'S BUTTONS, COCKLEBUR

Burdock is an ancient and versatile herb best known from the drink dandelion-and-burdock. Its roots are eaten by the Japanese as a vegetable for the dietary fiber they contain. Native to northern Europe, burdock is also found in Asia and North America. It is a perennial with a deep taproot, large arrow-shaped leaves, and thistlelike purple flowers that are surrounded by tiny hooks, so sticking to passing animals or to clothes.

PARTS USED: Leaves, seeds, root.
ACTIVE INGREDIENTS: Inulin and polyacetylenes in the root; lignans, including arctigenin; sesquiterpenes in the leaves; fixed oil; organic acids, including phenolic acids.
ACTIONS: Increases urine production; stimulates nutrition and elimination; stimulates the appetite; mildly sedative; antibacterial; laxative.
MEDICINAL USE: Most often used for skin diseases, particularly eczema and psoriasis. It is also given for gout, rheumatism, anorexia, and infective cystitis. In Chinese medicine, the root is given internally for rheumatism, gout, catarrh, and infective skin conditions such as syphilis, and is applied externally for hemorrhoids, sores, and swellings. The seeds are prescribed for psoriasis and to stimulate the stomach.
PREPARATIONS: Infusion, decoction, tincture.

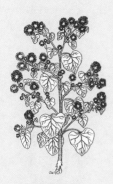

Arctium lappa

Arctostaphylos uva-ursi (Ericaceae)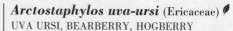
UVA URSI, BEARBERRY, HOGBERRY

Bearberry has been recognized as a diuretic in Europe since the Middle Ages, and its antibacterial properties were confirmed by German physicians in the 18th century. It grows throughout the northern hemisphere in the highlands of high latitudes and is found in North America, Europe, and Asia. The plant is low and creeping, with spatula-like leaves and small clusters of white or pink waxy flowers.

PARTS USED: Leaves collected in late summer.
ACTIVE INGREDIENTS: Hydroquinnones, including arbutin; iridoids; flavonoids, including quercitin; tannins; volatile oil.
ACTIONS: Increases urine production; antiseptic; astringent.
MEDICINAL USE: Given for cystitis and other inflammatory urinary tract conditions, and for painful urination.
PREPARATIONS: Infusion, tincture, tablets.

Argentite
ACANTHITE, SILVER SULFIDE

Argentite is the most important source of silver and can be so easily formed into a shape that it was originally used to make coins. Coins minted in Jachymov, Czechoslovakia, where it occurs naturally, were called Joachimsthalergulden, which is the origin of the word dollar.

PARTS USED: Silver, to make silver nitrate.
ACTIVE INGREDIENTS: Silver.
ACTIONS:: Caustic; antibacterial.
MEDICINAL USE: Silver nitrate is applied externally to warts and to disinfect the skin in orthodox medicine. It is also one of the key homeopathic remedies (*Argentum nitrate*) taken for dizziness, conjunctivitis, itching scalp, colic, gas and diarrhea, and for headaches, particularly when they are associated with fear or nervousness.
PREPARATIONS: Lotion, stick, homeopathic remedies.

Armoracia rusticana/Cochlearia armoracia (Cruciferae)
HORSERADISH

Long known as a condiment, which the herbalist Parkinson said, in 1640, was "too strong for tender and gentle [British] stomachs," horseradish is used by Germans as the culinary equivalent of mustard. Native to central and eastern Europe but naturalized in many temperate countries as a garden escapee, it has long tapering leaves growing from a deep taproot and bunches of white flowers in late summer.

PARTS USED: Freshly harvested root.
ACTIVE INGREDIENTS: Vitamin C; glucosinolates, mainly sinigrin, which combine with water when crushed, producing mustard oils; resin.
ACTIONS: Stimulant; induces sweating; increases urine production; antibacterial.

MEDICINAL USE: Used as a circulatory stimulant and applied externally for gout and rheumatism. The mustard oils are antibacterial, so horseradish is also used to treat lung infections.
PREPARATIONS: Poultice, syrup, tincture.
CAUTION: **Care is necessary with the poultice as the plant may cause blistering.**

Arnica montana (Compositae) 🌿
LEOPARD'S BANE, MOUNTAIN TOBACCO

Widely used across Europe by physicians as a remedy for bruises and wounds since the 16th century, arnica was claimed by Goethe to have saved his life after a serious fever. It is a perennial that sends up a rosette of small downy leaves in the first year. A tall stem with few leaves but large daisylike flowers rises in the second year.

PARTS USED: Flowers, root.
ACTIVE INGREDIENTS: Sesquiterpene lactones; flavonoids; methylated flavonoids; volatile oil containing thymol; arnicin (a bitter); mucilage.
ACTIONS: Counterirritant; promotes wound healing; dilates the blood vessels.
MEDICINAL USE: Applied externally on bruises and sprains when the skin is unbroken, on chilblains (sores due to exposure to cold), and for alopecia neurotica (hair loss due to anxiety). Used internally only in homeopathic doses (*Arnica*) for shock, pain, inflammation, epilepsy, and sea sickness. It irritates the digestive tract and kidneys if taken internally at higher than homeopathic doses.
PREPARATIONS: Tincture, cream, homeopathic remedies.

Arsenopyrite 🎲☠
IRON ARSENIC SULFITE, MISPICKEL

The main source of arsenic, arsenopyrite occurs across the world as clumps of silvery gray crystals that have, when struck, a strong odor of garlic. Arsenic is a good example of how a deadly poison can be medically useful, as it is now a commonly used homeopathic remedy.

PARTS USED: Extracted arsenic trioxide.
ACTIVE INGREDIENTS: Arsenic.
ACTIONS: Blood tonic; caustic.
MEDICINAL USE: Used homeopathically (*Arsenicum album*) for food poisoning, restlessness, anxiety, insomnia, headache, menstrual cramps, and psoriasis. Given in Chinese medicine as a blood purifier and tonic for anemia, skin diseases, and asthma. Arsenic trioxide was prescribed for skin diseases such as eczema in orthodox medicine. However, it is no longer recommended because of its toxicity.
PREPARATIONS: Powdered metal, homeopathic remedies.

Artemisia abrotanum (Compositae) 🌿
SOUTHERNWOOD, GARDE ROBE, LAD'S LOVE

Southernwood has been a garden plant since the Middle Ages, and women used to carry sprigs of the herb for the pungent odor,

which they hoped might keep them awake during church services. Today, the Italians use it as a culinary herb. It is native to southern Europe but has been naturalized in Britain and North America. A perennial shrub with finely divided, feathery leaves, it has tiny yellowish flowers in late summer.

PARTS USED: Dried leaves and flowering tops.
ACTIVE INGREDIENTS: Volatile oil with absinthol.
ACTIONS: Stimulates menstruation; bitter (digestive stimulant); antiseptic; kills and helps expel worms.
MEDICINAL USE: Given for absent or delayed menstruation, threadworms in children, and as a bitter in digestive and liver complaints.
PREPARATIONS: Infusion, tincture.

Artemisia absinthium (Compositae) 🌿
WORMWOOD, ABSINTHE, GREEN GINGER

An ancient household insecticide against clothes moths, wormwood has also been employed as a substitute for hops in brewing, as a liqueur (though the sale of absinthe is now outlawed), and as an antiseptic. Native to many parts of Europe, it is now naturalized in North America, growing freely on roadsides and wasteland. It is a perennial with firm leafy stems and leaves that are pale from thick downy hairs. Small yellow flowers appear in late summer.

PARTS USED: Dried leaves, flowering tops.
ACTIVE INGREDIENTS: Volatile oil containing thujone, azulene, bisabolene, and pinene; sesquiterpene lactones; flavonoids, including quercetin; phenolic acids; lignans.
ACTIONS: Bitter (digestive stimulant); stimulates the stomach; increases the flow of bile; anti-inflammatory; kills and helps expel worms.
MEDICINAL USE: Used for parasitic worms, anorexia, and gastritis (stomach inflammation). In Chinese medicine, a related species (sweet wormwood) is prescribed for summer colds, malaria, and chronic dysentery, and is also applied externally for scabies, abscesses, and eye disorders.
PREPARATIONS: Infusion, tincture.

Asarum canadense (Aristolochiaceae) 🌿
WILD GINGER, CANADIAN SNAKEROOT

Not a ginger, although it smells similar, *A. canadense* was used as a contraceptive by Native Americans and as a stimulant by the early colonists. A native of North America, it grows in moist woodlands. A fleshy root produces two kidney-shaped leaves and one brownish, bell-like flower.

PARTS USED: Root collected in autumn.
ACTIVE INGREDIENTS: Volatile oil; asarin; resin; bitter principle.
ACTIONS: Stimulant; increases urine production; relieves gas and colic; induces sweating.
MEDICINAL USE: Used in flatulent indigestion. Chinese doctors prescribe wild ginger for bad breath, cold symptoms, watery eyes, hearing defects, headache, and toothache.
PREPARATIONS: Infusion, finely ground as snuff.

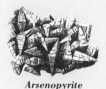

Arsenopyrite

Asclepias tuberosa (Asclepiadaceae)
PLEURISY ROOT, COLIC ROOT,
BUTTERFLY WEED

One of the most successful Native American remedies, it was used as a food, as a medicine, and in special ceremonies. When colonist doctors discovered it, they named it after the Greek god of medicine, Asklepios, because of its power to save lives. Indigenous to North America, it is a perennial, with spearlike leaves and yellow flowers in summer.

PARTS USED: Dried root.
ACTIVE INGREDIENTS: Glycosides, including ascelpiadin; flavonoids, including rutin, kaempferol, and quercitin; amino acids.
ACTIONS: Expectorant; induces sweating; reduces muscle tension and spasms; relieves gas and colic.
MEDICINAL USE: Given for respiratory conditions such as bronchitis, pneumonia, pleurisy, and flu, where it eases pain and difficult breathing.
PREPARATIONS: Infusion, tincture.
CAUTION: **Excess can cause vomiting and diarrhea, use with care.**

Atropa belladonna (Solanaceae)
BELLADONNA, DEADLY NIGHTSHADE,
DEVIL'S CHERRIES

Legend has it that the devil tends the growing plant, which contains one of the most medicinally used poisons. Duncan I of Scotland had Macbeth's soldiers drug an entire Danish army with a gift of a belladonna-laced liqueur, so they could be murdered in their comatose sleep. The name belladonna derives from the historic practice of Italian women using the plant to dilate their pupils, so making themselves more alluring. A native of southern Europe but also found in Asia, North Africa, and North America, it is a perennial with egg-shaped leaves. Purple, bell-shaped flowers are produced in summer, followed by highly poisonous black berries.

PARTS USED: Whole herb, dried root.
ACTIVE INGREDIENTS: Alkaloids, including hyoscyamine, hyoscine, and atropine; flavonoids.
ACTIONS: Narcotic; sedative; dilates the pupils, reduces muscle tension and spasms.
MEDICINAL USE: Given for severe intestinal, renal, or gallbladder colic, for excessive salivation or sweating, and for bronchial conditions such as asthma. It has also been used externally for rheumatic pain. Side effects include palpitations, raised blood pressure, and intense thirst. Used in homeopathy (*Belladonna*) for hot fevers, colds, headache, teething, sore throats, dry cough, abdominal pain, and convulsions. In orthodox medicine, belladonna preparations are still given for intestinal cramps, migraines, and arthritis.
PREPARATIONS: Infusion, tincture, cream, plasters, homeopathic remedies, pharmaceutical preparations.
CAUTION: **An overdose is dangerous and can even be lethal.**

Aurum
GOLD

The only explanation for gold's high value is that people felt the need to have an international currency. Gold achieved its status several thousand years ago, and its holders have always had a vested interest in maintaining its value. Gold's practical merits are that it is rare, never tarnishes, and is easily shaped. Just over half the gold not stored by individual countries is used in jewelry, a quarter is used in the electrical industry for its excellent conduction properties, and about 10 per cent is used in dentistry. Medicinally, gold is used as it is, in radioactive form, or as salts.

PARTS USED: Gold, gold salts.
ACTIVE INGREDIENTS: Gold.
ACTIONS: Radioactive; anti-inflammatory.
MEDICINAL USE: In orthodox medicine, radioactive gold is implanted into tissues as part of some radiation therapies for cancer and is sometimes given for rheumatoid arthritis, but its toxicity makes it a treatment of last resort. Nonradioactive gold is also used for rheumatoid arthritis in orthodox medicine in the form of salts such as sodium aurothiomalate. It is given homeopathically (*Aurum metallicum*) for conditions ranging from depression and arteriosclerosis to bone loss. Chinese physicians apply gold externally as a thin foil to bunions to reduce pain and inflammation.
PREPARATIONS: *Gold salts:* injections, tablets. *Radioactive gold:* in a gelatin suspension or water for injection, as granules for implants. *Homeopathic remedies. Gold foil.*

Avena sativa (Graminae)
OATS

Samuel Johnson defined oats as "a grain, which in England is generally given to horses, but in Scotland supports the people." Their origin is unknown, but oats have probably been eaten, if not cultivated, since neolithic times. Widely used in medicine, oats' traditional uses as a general nutritive and nerve restorative have been confirmed by recent experiments. The plant is an annual grass easily distinguished from wheat or barley by the loose head of grain and its papery covering.

PARTS USED: Flowering tops, grain.
ACTIVE INGREDIENTS: Alkaloids; flavonoids; protein; minerals, including silica and calcium.
ACTIONS: Restores the nerves; stimulant; supports the nutrition and tone of the nervous system.
MEDICINAL USE: Used for depression, melancholia, and for general debility involving the nervous system, such as occurs in shingles and multiple sclerosis. Prescribed in Ayurvedic medicine for opium withdrawal. Skin preparations containing oat extracts are still used in orthodox medicine for eczema and dry skin. If eaten in large amounts, oats may lower blood cholesterol levels.
PREPARATIONS: Groats, oatmeal, whole plant juice, tincture, over-the-counter skin preparations.

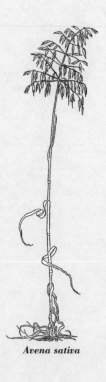
Avena sativa

Ballota nigra (Labiatae)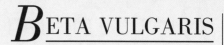
BLACK HOREHOUND

So foul smelling that cattle will not eat it, horehound derives its generic name from the Greek for reject. Culpeper linked horehound with the planet Mercury and recommended it be eaten with salt to "cure the bites of mad dogs." A native of temperate eastern Europe, it thrives in roadside ditches, hedgerows, and other moist places. It has square, hairy stems, creeping roots, heart-shaped, scallop-edged leaves, and small purple flowers from late summer.

PARTS USED: Flowering tops.
ACTIVE INGREDIENTS: Flavonoids.
ACTIONS: Sedative; suppresses nausea and vomiting; reduces muscle tension and spasms.
MEDICINAL USE: Given for nausea and vomiting, especially motion sickness and in pregnancy. It is also used for nervous dyspepsia (indigestion).
PREPARATIONS: Infusion, tincture.

Baptisia tinctoria (Leguminosae)
WILD INDIGO, RATTTLEWEED

This is not the source of the famous blue-jeans dye, but is a native to North America once used by Native Americans as a dye and for medicine. Wild indigo is a small perennial shrub with rounded, cloverlike leaves and bunches of small yellow flowers during late summer.

PARTS USED: Dried root.
ACTIVE INGREDIENTS: Isoflavones, including genistein and aptogenin; flavonoids; alkaloids, including cytisine; coumarins.
ACTIONS: Anti-infective; laxative; helps reduce fever; increases the flow of bile.
MEDICINAL USE: Given internally for infections and inflammation of the mouth, throat, or tonsils, inflammation of the lymphatic system, and as a douche for vaginal discharges. Externally, it is used on boils and ulcers, and for rheumatism.
PREPARATIONS: Decoction, tincture, cream.

Barite
HEAVY SPAR

The main ore for barium, barite takes its name from the Greek *barys*, meaning heavy. Barite occurs across the world and is transparent or translucent, comes in many shapes of crystal, and has a glassy or pearly appearance. It can be many colors, ranging from clear to yellow, blue, or brown, depending on the minerals it contains.

PARTS USED: Barium sulfate.
ACTIVE INGREDIENTS: Barium sulfate.
ACTIONS: Opaque to X-rays.
MEDICINAL USE: A barium meal enables a doctor to follow the progress of a liquid (barium sulfate suspension) or solid (bread soaked in barium suspension) down the digestive tract with X-rays to look for any changes in the digestive system.
PREPARATIONS: Suspension of barium sulfate.

Berberis aquifolium/Mahonia aquifolium (Berberidaceae)
OREGON GRAPE, HOLLY GRAPE

A common ornamental garden plant in temperate countries, it originated in the mountains between Oregon and British Columbia and has been introduced to other countries only since the mid-19th century. It is a tall shrub with large, hollylike, evergreen leaves, clusters of small, yellowish and strongly scented flowers, and bunches of smooth, dark purple berries.

PARTS USED: Root, rhizome.
ACTIVE INGREDIENTS: Alkaloids, including berberine, hydrastine, and oxycanthine.
ACTIONS: Laxative; suppresses nausea and vomiting; increases the flow of bile.
MEDICINAL USE: Used for inflammation of the stomach, gallbladder, or intestines, and for inflamed joints in rheumatic disease. Also given for skin complaints such as psoriasis and eczema.
PREPARATIONS: Decoction, tincture.
CAUTION: **Avoid during pregnancy.**

Berberis vulgaris (Berberidaceae)
COMMON BARBERRY, JAUNDICE BERRY, PIPRAGE

Indigenous to Europe, barberry became unpopular with farmers when it was discovered to be a host plant for the wheat rust fungus that decimated crops in the 19th century. It used to be cultivated for its fruit, which make delicious pickles and sweetmeats. A deciduous shrub, it has clusters of oval leaves and small yellow flowers from spring to midsummer, followed by oblong red berries with an acid taste.

PARTS USED: Bark of stem and root.
ACTIVE INGREDIENTS: Alkaloids, including berberine and oxycanthine; chelidonic acid; resin; tannins.
ACTIONS: Anti-inflammatory; antimicrobial; increases the flow of bile; suppresses nausea and vomiting; a digestive tonic.
MEDICINAL USE: Given for jaundice, gallstones, and digestive problems with liver involvement following drug or alcohol abuse. In Ayurvedic medicine, it is used against the parasitic diseases Leishmaniasis and malaria. In Chinese medicine, it is prescribed for dysentery and diarrhea.
PREPARATIONS: Decoction, tincture.
CAUTION: **Avoid during pregnancy.**

Beta vulgaris (Chenopodiaceae)
BEETROOT, RED BEET, WHITE BEET, SUGAR BEET

The red beet has been a prized vegetable since ancient Greece. Rich in sugars, it is made into wine as well as borscht. The white sugar beet was bred from the red form. Large, bright green leaves grow on stalks from a short stem, and a central spike with insignificant flowers appears in late summer. The swollen root varies from round to tapered like a carrot.

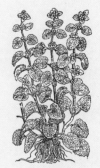

Ballota nigra

PARTS USED: Root.

ACTIVE INGREDIENTS: Sugars; an anthocyanin pigment betanin in red beet; the amino acid betaine in white beet; gums; resins.

ACTIONS: Stimulates the immune system; a liver restorative.

MEDICINAL USE: White beet is used in the treatment of jaundice and liver damage caused by drug or alcohol abuse. Red beet is given to enhance the body's resistance when debilitated by a chronic infectious disease. In Europe, beetroot is used against cancers.

PREPARATIONS: Fresh root, juice.

Betula pendula/B. alba/B. verrucosa
(Betulaceae) ✑
EUROPEAN WHITE BIRCH

The bark of the white birch tree has been used since mesolithic times as a paper and house construction material. Found throughout northern Europe, northern Asia, and North America, the white birch is a tall deciduous tree with a silvery white bark that peels easily into horizontal strips. The leaves are arrow-shaped with a serrated edge and the flowers are known as catkins.

PARTS USED: Bark, leaves.

ACTIVE INGREDIENTS: Flavonoids, mainly hyperoside, luteolin and quercetin; saponins; volatile oil containing betulin; resin; tannins.

ACTIONS: Anti-inflammatory; astringent; increases urine production; urinary disinfectant; increases the flow of bile; induces sweating.

MEDICINAL USE: Used in rheumatic and arthritic disease, and in active autoimmune diseases. Also prescribed for edema (swelling due to fluid accumulation), urinary tract infections, and kidney stones.

PREPARATIONS: Infusion, decoction, tincture, juice.

Bothrops jararaca

Bismuth ⊚

Found worldwide, the silvery white crystals of bismuth have a long history of medicinal use, but poor results and side effects such as anorexia and jaundice reduced bismuth's traditional applications. Now, however, it has been rediscovered and many products containing bismuth salts are still available.

PARTS USED: Bismuth, to make bismuth salts.

ACTIVE INGREDIENTS: Bismuth.

ACTIONS: Antibacterial; protects the lining of the stomach.

MEDICINAL USE: In orthodox medicine, bismuth and certain bismuth salts used to be given for syphilis but have since been superseded by antibiotics. Now, some salts such as bismuth subcitrate are used in preparations for indigestion and, since the discovery that peptic ulcers may be caused by the bacteria *Helicobacter pylori*, are being prescribed to treat peptic ulceration because they have antibacterial properties. Other bismuth salts are still applied externally for hemorrhoids.

PREPARATIONS: Liquid suspension, ointment, cream, suppositories, tablets.

Boswellia thurifera/B. carterii
(Burseraceae) ✑
FRANKINCENSE, OLIBANUM, MASTIC TREE

Once so highly esteemed that, along with myrrh and gold, it was presented to the Christ child, frankincense, with its familiar smell, accompanies Christian ceremonies throughout the world. It is native to East Africa and Arabia, where it is used by women as eye makeup and as a depilatory. A tall tree, it has leaves with up to ten pairs of opposite leaflets. The resin is tapped by cutting grooves in the trunk. It is then left to dry before being collected.

PARTS USED: Sap, resin.

ACTIVE INGREDIENTS: Volatile oil containing terpenes and sesquiterpenes; resin; gum.

ACTIONS: Antiseptic; stimulant.

MEDICINAL USE: Applied externally to wounds, and used as an inhalation in bronchitis and as a gargle for throat and mouth infections. Chinese physicians have prescribed it for leprosy and other skin infections, for amenorrhea and menstrual cramps, as a painkiller for abdominal pain, and as a cough suppressant.

PREPARATIONS: Powdered resin.

Bothrops jararaca ⚕
PIT VIPER

Like other pit vipers, this South American snake is not only venomous but quick to attack. It can grow to an alarming 4 feet long and is easily camouflaged in its grassland habitat by its olive-brown markings. It is extremely poisonous and therefore used medicinally to make an antidote for its own venom.

PARTS USED: Venom.

ACTIVE INGREDIENTS: Antivenin; teprotide.

ACTIONS: Lowers blood pressure.

MEDICINAL USE: A synthetic teprotide has been used in orthodox medicine to investigate high blood pressure. The venom of *Bothrops jararaca* is used to make an antidote.

PREPARATIONS: Injections.

Calculus bovis ⚕
CATTLE GALLSTONES, BEZOARS

The lumps of mineral salts, or gallstones, that occur in the gallbladders of many species of mammal are known as bezoars, which translates from Arabic as "against poison." Bezoars have had a semi-magical reputation and a long Eastern and Western history of medical use. The stones are oval-shaped, yellow, green, or brown in color, and brittle with a bitter taste. Their main ingredients are cholesterol and other fatty acids, amino acids, and minerals.

PARTS USED: Whole gallstones.

ACTIVE INGREDIENTS: Not known.

ACTIONS: Anticonvulsant; helps reduce fever; sedative; increases urine production.

MEDICINAL USE: Chinese and Unani physicians use

cattle bezoars, as Western medicine used to, for their effect on fevers, swollen sore throats, carbuncles, abscesses, other "hot" complaints, and also for spasms.

PREPARATIONS: Powder, pills.

CAUTION: Avoid during pregnancy.

Calendula officinalis (Compositae) 🌿
POT MARIGOLD

Found throughout the world as a garden plant, the marigold is also one of the most useful herbal remedies and has long been used in Indian, Arabic, and Greek medicine. Such large amounts are grown for medicinal use in the republic of Russia that it has earned the nickname of Russian penicillin. An annual, it has hairy, oblong leaves and large, yellow or orange, daisylike flowers from early summer until the first frosts.

PARTS USED: Flower heads, leaves.

ACTIVE INGREDIENTS: Triterpenes; carotenoids; saponins; flavonoids, including quercetin; rutin; volatile oil; resin; chlorogenic acid.

ACTIONS: Anti-inflammatory; antiseptic; antifungal; reduces muscle tension and spasms; promotes wound healing; stops bleeding from external wounds; stimulates menstruation.

MEDICINAL USE: Given internally for inflammation of the lymph nodes, mouth ulcers, a damaged or ulcerated stomach lining, and as a gargle for throat infections and oral thrush. Externally, it is applied to leg ulcers, hemorrhoids, anal fissures (small cracks), and eczema, as an eye lotion for conjunctivitis, and as a douche against vaginal thrush. Homeopathically, *Calendula* is prescribed for coughs, the common cold, fever, wounds, and chronic infections.

PREPARATIONS: Infusion, tincture, cream, homeopathic remedies.

Cannabis sativa (Cannabaceae) 🌿
MARIJUANA, GANJA, HEMP, HASHISH

Known in Indian and Chinese herbals for more than 1,500 years, cannabis was brought to Europe by Napoleon after his Egyptian exploits. Popular as a mild but illegal drug, it is also useful as a source of fibers for making sacking, string, and rope. Cultivated in China, India, and southern Russia, the wild plants are sometimes found in temperate Europe and North America. An annual, cannabis has leaves of long, deeply serrated leaflets. Separate male and female plants bear small, inconspicuous flowers in late summer.

PARTS USED: Leaf, resin, seeds.

ACTIVE INGREDIENTS: A resin containing over 60 components called cannabinoids; volatile oil; flavonoids.

ACTIONS: Reduces muscle tension and spasms; relieves pain; intoxicant; a cerebral sedative.

MEDICINAL USE: Used herbally for neuralgia, spasmodic cough, and migraine. Prescribed by doctors for the relief of nausea and vomiting in cancer patients on chemotherapy, and also for glaucoma. A synthetic cannabinoid (nabilone) is

also given in orthodox medicine for the same purpose. Chinese medicine uses the seeds as a tonic, laxative, and emollient.

PREPARATIONS: Resin, dried leaf, tincture, nabilone capsules.

CAUTION: Possession of cannabis is illegal in the United States and Canada.

Capsella bursa-pastoris (Cruciferae) 🌿
SHEPHERD'S PURSE, MOTHER'S HEART, STRANGURY, COCOWORT, ST. JAMES' WEED, SHEPHERD'S HEART

The distinctive heart-shaped fruit of *C. bursa-pastoris* resembles the purses that people in medieval Europe used to hang from their belts, hence the common name of shepherd's purse. Native to Europe, it has spread to all temperate parts of the world, and has long been popular in traditional medicine for stopping bleeding. It is a low-growing annual herb with irregular, pale green, hairy leaves, and inconspicuous white flowers throughout the year.

PARTS USED: Leaves.

ACTIVE INGREDIENTS: Flavonoids; polypeptides; fumaric and bursic acids; tryamine, choline, and acetylcholine; glucosinolates.

ACTIONS: Prevents hemorrhage; a urinary antiseptic; mildly increases urine production.

MEDICINAL USE: Given for many forms of bleeding, from nosebleeds and internal bleeding to excessive menstrual blood loss. Also used in urinary tract infections and for kidney stones.

PREPARATIONS: Infusion, tincture.

Capsicum (Solanaceae) 🌿
CHILE PEPPERS

Hot chiles, natives of Africa, the Caribbean, and South America, are widely used in spicy foods; cayenne pepper and Tabasco are chile-based seasonings. The existence of hot chiles was recorded by Columbus's doctor on his second voyage to the West Indies in 1494. They are hotter than the larger Indian chiles and are relatives of the sweet pepper, or capsicum, from which the seasoning paprika is made.

PARTS USED: Fruit.

ACTIVE INGREDIENTS: A phenolic compound, capsaicin; carotenoids; saponins known as capsicidins; flavonoids; volatile oil.

ACTIONS: Increases blood flow; induces sweating; reduces muscle tension and spasms; stimulates blood flow to the skin; relieves gas and colic; counterirritant; antiseptic.

MEDICINAL USE: Widely used in conditions where reduced blood circulation is a factor, including digestive debility, flatulent colic, and reduced peripheral (local) circulation. Applied externally for joint inflammation, unbroken chilblains (sores that result from exposure to cold), and lumbago (lower back pain).

PREPARATIONS: Tincture, cream, powder.

CAUTION: Use only in small doses to avoid irritating the stomach or burning the skin.

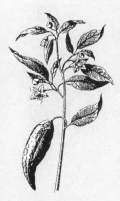

Capsicum

Carbon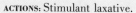

COAL, BITUMINOUS COAL

Coal, the fossil we take for granted, is transformed over many millions of years from compressed plants to a hard, black mineral. The main kind of coal used as a medicinal source is known as bituminous coal. The destructive distillation of coal gives rise to coal gas, various grades of tar, and coke. More than 200 substances can be made from coal tars. Some of these substances form the basis of the most criticized food colorings and others are useful medicinally.

PARTS USED: Coal tar.
ACTIVE INGREDIENTS: Coal tar.
ACTIONS: Alleviates itching; weak antiseptic; kills skin cells.
MEDICINAL USE: Prescribed in orthodox medicine to combat skin complaints such as psoriasis, dandruff, and eczema.
PREPARATIONS: Over-the-counter ointment, paint, paste, solution, gel, cream, and shampoo.

Carica papaya (Curcurbitaceae)

PAPAYA, PAW PAW, MELON TREE

One of the most fragrant of tropical fruits, it is eaten green as a vegetable or ripe as a fruit. Native to South America but now cultivated throughout the tropics, this tall herbaceous plant has large, deeply divided leaves. The fruit is oblong, ripens to yellow with deep yellow-orange flesh, and has a central cavity filled with small black seeds.

PARTS USED: White latex from fruit, fresh leaves.
ACTIVE INGREDIENTS: Alkaloid carpaine in leaves; enzyme papain from latex.
ACTIONS: Kills and helps expel worms; dissolves protein in dead skin; stimulates the stomach; promotes wound healing.
MEDICINAL USE: Given for indigestion and gastritis (stomach inflammation), and effective against threadworms and roundworms. Also applied externally to deep, slow-healing wounds; fresh leaves can be wrapped directly around wounds.
PREPARATIONS: Powdered enzyme, tablets.

Cassia acutifolia/C. senna
(Leguminosae)

ALEXANDRIAN SENNA

The first records of senna's medicinal use come from Arabian physicians who imported material through Alexandria, from which one of the common names derives. Senna now provides the main ingredient of many pharmaceutical laxatives. A small shrubby plant with leaves divided into opposite leaflets, it has small yellow flowers that give way to flat, curved pods, each of which contains six seeds.

PARTS USED: Leaves, pods.
ACTIVE INGREDIENTS: Anthraquinone glycosides, including sennosides A, B, C, D, palmidin A, aloe-emodin, and rhein; kaempferol; mucilage.

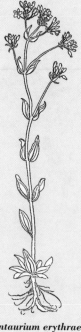

Centaurium erythraea

ACTIONS: Stimulant laxative.
MEDICINAL USE: Widely used in many systems of medicine to treat constipation due to lack of tone or contraction of the bowel, but it should not be used for spastic constipation or colitis (an inflammatory condition of the intestines).
PREPARATIONS: Powdered leaves, infusion, tablets, tincture, over-the-counter preparations.

Caulophyllum thalictroides
(Berberidaceae)

BLUE COHOSH, BEECHDROPS, SQUAWROOT

Native Americans have a long tradition of using blue cohosh to ease the pain of childbirth, and it was one of the medicines brought to Europe during the 19th century. Native to North America, it grows wild in moist mountain valleys, and has a tortuous branching rootstock, lobed leaflets, and small, yellow-green, six-petalled flowers in early summer.

PARTS USED: Root.
ACTIVE INGREDIENTS: Steroidal saponins, including caulosaponin; alkaloids, including caulophylline.
ACTIONS: Anti-inflammatory; a strong expectorant; stimulates menstruation; reduces muscle tension and spasms; increases uterine muscle tone.
MEDICINAL USE: Prescribed mainly for uterine conditions, including amenorrhea, menstrual cramps, and pain associated with pelvic inflammatory disease or fibroids. It is also used for rheumatism.
PREPARATIONS: Decoction, tincture, extract.
CAUTION: **Avoid during pregnancy until labor has actually started.**

Centaurium erythraea/Erythaea centaurium (Gentianaceae)

CENTAURY, RED CENTAURY, FILWORT

The mythical centaur Chironia, who was skilled with herbal medicine, cured a poisoned arrow wound with centaury, hence its name. A classic bitter herb, it has a long tradition as a wound healer and curer of infections. Native to Europe and North Africa, it is an annual with pale green, shiny, spear-shaped leaves and clusters of red, five-petalled flowers in late summer.

PARTS USED: Leaves, stem.
ACTIVE INGREDIENTS: Glycosides known as secoiroids, including sweroside and gentiopicrin; alkaloids, including gentianine and gentioflavine; xanthones; phenolic acids; triterpenes, including sitosterol, campesterol, and stigmasterol.
ACTIONS: Bitter (digestive stimulant); stimulates the stomach; tonic.
MEDICINAL USE: Given for anorexia and indigestion, particularly if the liver or gallbladder are weak.
PREPARATIONS: Infusion, tincture.

Cephaelis ipecacuanha (Rubiaceae)

IPECACUANHA ROOT, MATTO GROSSO

This plant is still harvested from the tropical forests of Brazil, where it is native. Its medicinal value was recorded first by a

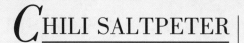

Portuguese friar who lived in Brazil around 1600, and it was brought to Europe 70 years later. It became so popular as a treatment for dysentery that the French government bought a formula of the herb from the doctor Helvetius, who was selling his own patent medicine. A perennial with a fibrous root and oval leaves, it produces clusters of small, mauve flowers in the autumn, followed by small, purple berries.

PARTS USED: Root.
ACTIVE INGREDIENTS: Alkaloids, especially emetine, cephaeline, and protoemetine; tannins; glycosides; saponins.
ACTIONS: Expectorant; causes vomiting; kills protozoa.
MEDICINAL USE: Prescribed by herbalists and in orthodox medicine for chest coughs such as bronchitis, and also given as an emetic to cause vomiting, especially in drug overdose where the stomach needs to be emptied immediately. As a herb, it has been used against amebic dysentery. Used in homeopathy (*Ipecac*) for coughing associated with nausea and vomiting, and for morning sickness.
PREPARATIONS: Decoction, tincture, in proprietary cough medicines, homeopathic remedies.
CAUTION: **Large doses are an irritant to the whole intestine and should be taken only on the advice of a qualified practitioner.**

Cetraria islandica (Parmeliaceae)
ICELAND MOSS

Despite its common name, this moss is a lichen, growing on stony, barren ground in high latitudes in northern Europe, Iceland, the North American tundra, and even Antarctica. It contains up to 70 per cent "lichen starch" and has long been used as an emergency food in desolate places. A branched and curly perennial plant, it is gray-brown or olive on top and paler with tiny white spots underneath.

PARTS USED: Whole lichen.
ACTIVE INGREDIENTS: Bitter acids, including cetraric, fumarprotocetraric, and lichesteric; mucilaginous polysaccharides, including isolichenin and lichenin.
ACTIONS: Expectorant; soothes internal body surfaces; suppresses nausea and vomiting; antibiotic; nutritive.
MEDICINAL USE: Given for gastritis (stomach inflammation), indigestion with vomiting, catarrh, and bronchitis.
PREPARATIONS: Decoction, cold infusion, tincture, tablets, in proprietary cough medicines.

Chamaelirium luteum (Liliaceae)
RATTLESNAKE ROOT, DEVIL'S-BIT, FAIRY-WAND

Rattlesnake root is a particularly useful bequest from the Native Americans' detailed knowledge of those herbs helpful for disorders of the female reproductive organs. Growing in wet places in the southeastern

United States, this perennial has spear-shaped leaves, a small round rhizome, and tiny green-white flowers in late summer.

PARTS USED: Rhizome.
ACTIVE INGREDIENTS: Saponins; glycosides, including chamaelirin and helonin.
ACTIONS: Increases uterine muscle tone; increases urine production; kills and helps expel worms.
MEDICINAL USE: Used for female reproductive tract problems, such as amenorrhea, menstrual cramps, threatened miscarriage, morning sickness, and for certain forms of female infertility.
PREPARATIONS: Infusion, tincture.

Chelidonium majus (Papaveraceae)
GREATER CELANDINE, TETTERWORT

An ancient liver remedy mentioned in many of the great herbals, *celandine* derives from the Greek for "swallows" because it starts flowering when they arrive and stops when they leave. It is native to Europe but has been introduced throughout the temperate world. A perennial, it has deeply cut, pale green leaves that are thin and hairy, and a stem that oozes rich orange latex if cut or broken. Small clusters of delicate, bright yellow flowers are produced all summer, followed by thin pods.

PARTS USED: Whole herb.
ACTIVE INGREDIENTS: Alkaloids, including berberine, chelamine, and chelidonine; saponins; choline.
ACTIONS: Increases the flow of bile; increases urine production; reduces muscle tension and spasms.
MEDICINAL USE: Given internally for jaundice, gallstones, and gallbladder disease. Applied externally for eczema, verrucas, and warts. It has also been used to remove cataracts. Used in homeopathy (*Chelidonium*) for nervous headache, nausea, and vomiting. Chinese physicians prescribe it as a painkiller, cough suppressant, and anti-inflammatory for bronchitis and whooping cough.
PREPARATIONS: Infusion, tincture, homeopathic remedies.
CAUTION: **Only use under the guidance of a qualified practitioner.**

Chili saltpeter
SALTPETER, SODIUM NITRATE

Named from the Latin for "salt of the rock," this white crystalline substance is an important source of iodine. It is also a long-established preservative for curing meat, but its safety is in doubt. Iodine forms part of the hormone thyroxine that regulates the thyroid gland, which in turn controls the body's whole rate of activity. Insufficient iodine leads to a lack of thyroxine, and a slowing down of the body's metabolism. This can lead to swelling of the thyroid gland, a goiter, as it attempts to redress the balance. In recent years, the addition of iodine to table salt has been widely and successfully used to prevent goiter. Chinese physicians realized the link between iodine

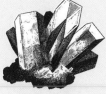

Chili saltpeter

and the thyroid gland about 2,000 years ago and treated goiter with burnt seaweed, which is rich in iodine.

PARTS USED: Iodine.
ACTIVE INGREDIENTS: Iodine.
ACTIONS: Nutrient; antiseptic.
MEDICINAL USE: Iodine is widely used in disinfectants. In orthodox medicine, iodine compounds are prescribed with antithyroid drugs for people with overactive thyroid glands prior to thyroid surgery, and are also used for the prevention and treatment of iodine deficiency.
PREPARATIONS: Solution, tincture, ointment, paint.

Chondrus crispus (Gigartinaceae)
IRISH MOSS, CARRAGEEN, PEARL MOSS

A red algae that flourishes in the cool waters of the North Atlantic, carrageen is used as an emulsifier in a wide range of foods. It comes in many forms, having anything from fan-shaped to ribbonlike fronds. Dried, the fronds are yellow-brown and translucent.

PARTS USED: Dried plant.
ACTIVE INGREDIENTS: Gel-forming polysaccharides known as carrageens.
ACTIONS: Soothes internal body surfaces; cough suppressant; nutritive.
MEDICINAL USE: Given for indigestion associated with nausea and heartburn, gastritis (stomach inflammation), bronchitis, and irritable cough. It is also used as an emulsifier (enabling water and oil to mix) in medicines such as cod liver oil.
PREPARATIONS: Infusion.

Chromite
CHROMIUM ORE

The only ore of chromium, brownish black chromite is found across the world. The metal chromium was only recognized as essential to man in the 1960s. The first convincing evidence came from experiments showing that rats fed a chromium-deficient diet develop symptoms similar to those of diabetes. Other tests have shown that people with diabetes tolerate sugar better when given extra chromium. However, because there are no clear-cut deficiency symptoms, no one is sure how much we need.

PARTS USED: Chromium salts.
ACTIVE INGREDIENTS: Chromium.
ACTIONS: Nutrient.
MEDICINAL USE: Supplements are taken to ensure an adequate chromium intake when ability to absorb nutrients is reduced, such as in cystic fibrosis, or when need may be higher, such as in diabetes.
PREPARATIONS: Tablets, capsules.

Cimicifuga racemosa (Ranunculaceae)
BLACK COHOSH, BLACK SNAKEROOT, RATTLEROOT, BUGBANE

Native Americans claimed this herb cured the poisonous bites of rattlesnakes and also used it to ease the pain of menstruation and childbirth. Early settlers soon learned of

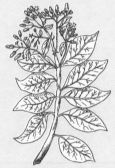

Cinchona succirubra

these benefits and the herb was introduced to European medicine in the 19th century. Native to North America, where it grows in open woodland, it is perennial with a black root, serrated leaflets, and strong-smelling, creamy white flowers in summer.

PARTS USED: Root and rhizome collected in autumn.
ACTIVE INGREDIENTS: Ranunculin, which converts to anemonin; triterpene glycosides, including actein, cimifugine, and racemoside; isoflavones.
ACTIONS: Anti-inflammatory; sedative; reduces muscle tension and spasms; stimulates nutrition and elimination; dilates the blood vessels.
MEDICINAL USE: Given for muscular rheumatism, neuralgia, muscle cramps, and other inflammatory conditions associated with pain such as menstrual cramps. Also used to treat leukorrhea (excessive pale white vaginal discharge) and the paroxysmal coughing of bronchitis or whooping cough. Related species (*C. simplex* and *C. foetida*) are used in Chinese medicine for headaches and certain fevers.
PREPARATIONS: Decoction, tincture.
CAUTION: High doses are dangerous, use only on the advice of a qualified practitioner, and avoid during pregnancy.

Cinchona succirubra (Rubiaceae)
PERUVIAN BARK, JESUIT'S BARK, QUININE TREE

The Spanish learned of the power of quinine from the Peruvian Indians when they invaded South America. The Jesuits appear to be the first to have used it as a fever medicine in Europe, and it soon became the renowned preventive and cure for malaria. A perennial tree native to the jungles of the west coast of South America, it is now cultivated for medicines in India, East Africa, and the East Indies. It grows to 80 feet, and has egg-shaped leaves and clusters of small crimson flowers.

PARTS USED: Bark.
ACTIVE INGREDIENTS: Quinoline alkaloids, including quinine, quinidine, and cinchonine; glycosides; tannins; quinic acid.
ACTIONS: Antimalarial; astringent; reduces or prevents fever; stimulates digestion; reduces muscle tension and spasms.
MEDICINAL USE: Used to prevent and treat malaria. Also given for liver conditions associated with an enlarged spleen, anorexia, indigestion, hyperchlorhydria (excessive stomach acid production), cramps, myalgia (muscle pain), and fevers with excessive temperature. It has also been used to help prevent flu. In orthodox medicine, the active ingredient quinine is prescribed as an antimalarial and for muscle cramps, and is in several over-the-counter painkilling and cold remedies. Quinidine is given for certain types of cardiac arrhythmias (irregular heart beats).
PREPARATIONS: Decoction, tincture, pharmaceutical tablets, and injections.
CAUTION: Large doses should be avoided.

Cinnabaris 🎲
CINNABAR, QUICKSILVER, MERCURIC SULFIDE

Found throughout the world, cinnabar is the only important mercury-containing ore. Its dramatic crimson color first attracted man in ancient times, when it was collected to make the dye we call vermilion. But it was the Romans who discovered how to extract its mercury. Mercury's poisonous nature did not stop its frequent use in futile medicines until the 20th century, and it is still used in close proximity to man, for example, in thermometers, disinfectants, and fungicides.

PARTS USED: Mercuric sulfide.
ACTIVE INGREDIENTS: Mercury.
ACTIONS: Reduces muscle tension and spasms; sedative.
MEDICINAL USE: Although mercury is so toxic that its medicinal use in the West has greatly dwindled, most of us have mercury amalgam fillings in our teeth. The safety of this practice has recently been challenged. Chinese physicians give cinnabar to sedate and calm both physically- and emotionally-caused palpitations, and apply it as a powder for mouth ulcers, sore throats, and carbuncles. *Mercurius solubilis* is given homeopathically for mouth and throat sores, and for infected swellings such as tonsillitis.
PREPARATIONS: Powder, pills, homeopathic remedies.

Cinnamomum zeylanicum (Lauraceae) 🍃
CINNAMON

One of the spices revered in the Bible, it was brought to Europe in the 17th century by the Portuguese, who invaded Sri Lanka just to obtain supplies. The spice comes from the bark of the plant and is sold in lengths of rolled bark called quills. Now cultivated throughout the tropics, the cinnamon tree grows to 30 feet, has a thick bark, leathery leaves, and small flowers that hang in loose bunches.

PARTS USED: Inner bark of shoots.
ACTIVE INGREDIENTS: Volatile oil containing cinnamaldehyde, cinnamyl acetate and alcohol, and eugenol; tannins; coumarin.
ACTIONS: Reduces muscle tension and spasms; relieves gas and colic; stimulates the appetite; astringent.
MEDICINAL USE: Given for flatulent indigestion and colic, anorexia, infantile diarrhea, the common cold, and flu. Chinese and Ayurvedic medicine prescribe it for stomach and liver conditions.
PREPARATIONS: Infusion, tincture.

Clupeiformes species 🐟
HERRING FAMILY

Oil from the flesh of herrings and other oily fish is rich in essential fatty acids. Research into the oil and its extraction began in the 1960s, prompted by the surprising rate of heart disease among Eskimos, which is one of the lowest in the world despite their high dietary fat intake. It is now believed that the essential fatty acids in fish flesh oil are protective against heart disease. Herring is the best source, along with mackerel and salmon. Herring has a longstanding folk reputation for its health value, and whole fish provide concentrated nourishment in the form of protein, B vitamins, essential fatty acids, vitamin E, iron, and zinc.

PARTS USED: Flesh.
ACTIVE INGREDIENTS: Omega-3 long chain polyunsaturated fatty acids, including EPA (eicosapentaenoic acid) and DHA (docosahexaenoic acid).
ACTIONS: Reduces blood lipid levels and helps to prevent blood clotting; anti-inflammatory; boosts immune function; lowers blood pressure.
MEDICINAL USE: Prescribed by doctors for hyperlipidemia (high blood cholesterol and fat levels), to prevent atherosclerosis (the clogging of arteries with cholesterol deposits), coronary thrombosis (a heart attack due to a blood clot blocking a coronary artery), and other thromboses such as strokes. There is also increasing interest in the use of fish flesh oils to lower blood pressure, for psoriasis, eczema, and arthritis, and to boost the immune system.
PREPARATIONS: Capsules, or 2 or 3 large, e.g. 8-ounce, portions of herring per week.

Cnicus benedictus/Carduus benedictus (Compositae) 🍃
ST. BENEDICT THISTLE, HOLY THISTLE, BLESSED THISTLE

The common names of *C. benedictus* reflect its veneration as a cure of the plague. Shakespeare said in *Much Ado About Nothing* that "It is the only thing for a qualm," but its more recent fame is due to its use in the liqueur Benedictine. A native of southern Europe, it is naturalized in the United States and cultivated in many other countries. It is a thistlelike annual with spear-shaped toothed leaves with a spine on each tooth, and flower heads covered in sharp, bristly scales.

PARTS USED: Flowering herb.
ACTIVE INGREDIENTS: Bitter glycosides, including cnicin; alkaloids; volatile oil; tannins; mucilage.
ACTIONS: Astringent; bitter (digestive stimulant); prevents hemorrhage; induces sweating.
MEDICINAL USE: Used internally in the treatment of anorexia, indigestion, sluggish digestion, and infectious gastritis (stomach inflammation), and applied externally to wounds and ulcers. Many related thistles are used medicinally; for example, Chinese physicians prescribe tiger thistle to stop internal bleeding and for high blood pressure.
PREPARATIONS: Infusion, tincture.

Cochlearia officinalis (Cruciferae) 🍃
SCURVY GRASS, SPOONWORT

Long before vitamin C was discovered, scurvy was a recognized disease known to occur whenever fruit and vegetables were scarce. These shortages happened in big

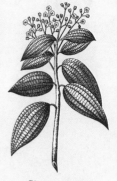

Cinnamomum zeylanicum

cities, during famine, and on sea voyages. Even then scurvy grass was known to cure the symptoms of scurvy, but it was only recently discovered that the plant is as rich in vitamin C as fresh oranges. A native of marshy European coastal lands, it is a small annual with thick, fleshy, egg-shaped leaves and clusters of white flowers in summer.

PARTS USED: Leaves.
ACTIVE INGREDIENTS: Glucosinolates; vitamin C.
ACTIONS: Prevents scurvy; promotes wound healing.
MEDICINAL USE: It was used in the past to treat scurvy, and is now applied externally to slow-healing wounds and ulcers.
PREPARATIONS: Fresh herb, infusion.

Coffea arabica (Rubiaceae) 🍃
COFFEE

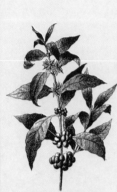

Coffea arabica

Coffee has been viewed variously as panacea or poison throughout its history. However, remarks about its dangers have often met with comments such as Voltaire's: "I have been poisoning myself for more than eighty years and I am not yet dead." A native of Ethiopia, coffee is named after the province of Caffa, where the fruit used to be chewed as a stimulant. It was introduced to Europe via Arabia in about 1650, and plants were also taken to the Far East and South America, which now supplies most of the world's crop. The tree has shiny, dark green, oval leaves and small, white flowers that turn into green berries. These ripen to a deep red and contain the coffee beans.

PARTS USED: Seeds, leaves.
ACTIVE INGREDIENTS: Caffeine; tannins; fats; sugars.
ACTIONS: Stimulant; increases urine production; antinarcotic; suppresses nausea and vomiting.
MEDICINAL USE: Used as a stimulant in narcotic poisoning to stop sleep. A common ingredient of many pharmaceutical painkilling preparations:, added to increase their effect. In homeopathic doses (*Coffea*), it is given for sleeplessness due to mental activity, tension, and anxiety.
PREPARATIONS: Infusion of roasted beans or dried leaves, tablets, injections, homeopathic remedies.

Cola vera (Sterculiaceae) 🍃
COLA TREE, GOORA NUT

Many people throughout West Africa, South America, and Asia chew cola nuts before meals to promote digestion; regular chewers can be recognized by their red lips and teeth. An evergreen, the cola tree is native to West Africa but was taken to the West Indies and South America by slaves and to India and Sri Lanka by traders. The nuts, which contain the seeds, are white when harvested but turn a red-brown when dried.

PARTS USED: Seeds.
ACTIVE INGREDIENTS: Alkaloids, especially caffeine and theobromine; tannins; red pigment.
ACTIONS: Central nervous system stimulant;

increases urine production; general stimulant.
MEDICINAL USE: Used as a tonic to stimulate the appetite and alleviate tiredness.
PREPARATIONS: Tablets, seeds, tincture, powder.

Commiphora molmol/C. myrrha (Burseraceae) 🍃
MYRRH, MIRRA, DIDTHIN, GUM MYRRH TREE

There are many Old Testament references to myrrh, and its name is thought to derive from the legend of Myrrh, whom the gods turned into a tree to protect her from her father's anger at discovering he had been tricked into incest. A shrub with gnarled branches and small, three-petalled leaves, myrrh is native to the driest parts of Northeast Africa and Arabia, and Somalia is the main source of the drug.

PARTS USED: Oleo-gum resin from the stems.
ACTIVE INGREDIENTS: Volatile oil containing heerabolene, canidene, and eugenol; resin consisting of commiphoric acids, commiphorinic acid, and heerabomyrrhols; gums consisting of aribinose, galactose, and xylose.
ACTIONS: Stimulant; expectorant; antiseptic; anti-inflammatory; promotes wound healing.
MEDICINAL USE: Most used in mouthwashes for mouth ulcers, inflamed gums, and sore throats. It is also given internally for lung infections associated with colds and catarrhal congestion, and applied externally to boils, wounds, and abrasions. Prescribed in Ayurvedic medicine to stimulate menstruation and as an alterative (to hasten the renewal of body tissues), and in Chinese medicine for wounds, amenorrhea, menstrual cramps, and rheumatism.
PREPARATIONS: Tincture, tablets, tooth powder.

Concha ostrea ⚕
OYSTER SHELL

Found throughout the world, the oyster shell is a grayish color on the outside and pearly white on the inside. Like other shells of bivalve shellfish – and several are used in similar ways – the oyster shell consists mainly of calcium salts. As well as being used as a calcium supplement, oyster shell has many diverse applications in Chinese, Unani, and homeopathic medicine.

PARTS USED: Shell.
ACTIVE INGREDIENTS: Calcium carbonate; calcium phosphate; iodine.
ACTIONS: Astringent; sedative; neutralizes excess stomach acid.
MEDICINAL USE: Given in Chinese and Unani medicine as a calcium supplement, for instance to strengthen the gums and teeth, and also for indigestion, high blood pressure, restlessness, insomnia, tinnitus (ringing in the ears), night sweats, uterine disorders, and after fevers. The homeopathic medicine, *Calcarea carbonica*, is prescribed for a range of conditions, from headaches and dizziness to night sweats and acute eye infections.
PREPARATIONS: Powder, tablets, homeopathic remedies.

Convallaria majalis (Liliaceae)
LILY OF THE VALLEY

The apothecaries of the Middle Ages recognized the value of this herb in "disorders of the heart and vital spirits." Its renown in the treatment of fainting, poor memory, "convulsions of all kinds and swimming in the head" may also stem from its beneficial effect on the heart and hence the blood circulation to the brain. A native of Europe, North America, and northern Asia, it has an underground stem, oval leaves, and fragrant, bell-shaped, white flowers in spring.

PARTS USED: Flowering tops, root.
ACTIVE INGREDIENTS: Glycosides, including convallarin, convallatoxin, and convalloside; flavonoids; asparagin.
ACTIONS: Improves the heart's pumping action; increases urine production.
MEDICINAL USE: It has a similar action to *Digitalis* (see p. 99) but is less toxic. Used in cardiac failure, as it helps the heart to beat more efficiently. The diuretic effect also helps to relieve edema (swelling due to fluid retention) associated with cardiac failure. In Chinese medicine, related species are used as a tonic.
PREPARATIONS: Tincture.

Coriandrum sativum (Umbelliferae)
CORIANDER, CILANTRO

An ancient herb that has been cultivated for at least 3,000 years, it is indigenous to Italy but now grows throughout the world and has become an established ingredient in traditional cookery in Peru, India, and the Middle East. Its name derives from the Greek for bug because of the insectlike smell of its leaves. An annual, it has many leaflets and small white flowers in summer, followed by spherical fruit.

PARTS USED: Fruit.
ACTIVE INGREDIENTS: Volatile oil containing coriandrol (55–74 percent), borneol, linalol, camphor, geraniol, limonene, and terpinene; flavonoids, including quercetin, kaempferol, and apigenin; coumarins; phenolic acids, including caffeic and chlorogenic.
ACTIONS: Aromatic; relieves gas and colic; reduces muscle tension and spasms.
MEDICINAL USE: Used largely as a carminative to relieve flatulence. Given in Ayurvedic medicine for urinary tract infections, skin conditions, burns, sore throats, indigestion, and allergies, and by Chinese physicians for measles, stomachache, and nausea.
PREPARATIONS: Powdered fruit, tincture, infusion.

Crataegus oxycanthoides/C. laevigata (Rosaceae)
HAWTHORN, ENGLISH HAWTHORN, WHITETHORN

Hawthorn flowers are reputed to have magical properties, such as causing a death in the family if they are taken into the home. The plant is also said to have been the source of Christ's crown of thorns. It is one of the most useful herbal heart remedies. Native to Europe, North Africa, and western Asia, this shrub or small tree grows to 30 feet and has dark green leaves. Clusters of white flowers appear from early to midsummer, followed by red berries in the autumn.

PARTS USED: Flowers, leaves, fruit.
ACTIVE INGREDIENTS: Flavonoids, including rutin, quercitin, and vitexin; procyanidine; phenolic acids; trimethylamine; ascorbic acid; tannins.
ACTIONS: Dilates the blood vessels of the heart and outlying parts of the body; improves the heart's pumping action; controls both high and low blood pressure; slows down a fast heartbeat.
MEDICINAL USE: Given to improve blood flow to the heart and the efficiency of the heart's pumping action in heart failure, to improve local circulation and intermittent claudication (pain in the calves caused by spasm in the blood vessels supplying the leg muscles), for Raynaud's disease, to lower high blood pressure, and for angina. Ayurvedic medicine prescribes it for similar purposes. Chinese physicians use it for indigestion, menstrual cramps, and diarrhea.
PREPARATIONS: Infusion, tincture.

Crotalus horridus
RATTLESNAKE

This pit viper of North America is so named because of the horny, flat rings of its tail, which rattle when vibrated as it attacks. The venom from its bite is sometimes fatal.

PARTS USED: Venom.
ACTIVE INGREDIENTS: Not known.
ACTIONS: Not known.
MEDICINAL USE: Given homeopathically (*Crotalus*) for swelling and pain that is worse with pressure.
PREPARATIONS: Homeopathic remedies.

Cuprum
COPPER

Occurring naturally in many parts of the world, copper is one of the minerals essential to the human body, being needed for the formation of red blood cells and for bone growth. Copper is also thought to be involved in the formation of melanin (skin pigment), and in the production of vital cellular proteins known as RNA. Certain processing reduces food's copper content; rich food sources include shellfish, liver, wheat germ, whole-grain cereals, Brazil nuts, malted products, and cocoa.

PARTS USED: Copper.
ACTIVE INGREDIENTS: Copper.
ACTIONS: Nutrient, if a deficiency exists.
MEDICINAL USE: In orthodox medicine, copper supplements, usually in the form of copper sulfate, are given for copper deficiencies, to babies suffering from Menke's syndrome (an inherited inability to absorb copper in the uterus), to offset loss of copper due to drugs such

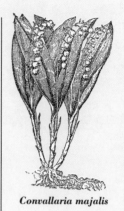

Convallaria majalis

as penicillamine, and in some forms of anemia. Copper also has a contraceptive effect and is included in some intrauterine contraceptive devices. Copper bracelets are worn as a folk remedy by many arthritis sufferers in the hope that some of the copper may be absorbed through the skin and have an anti-inflammatory effect. In homeopathy, as *Cuprum metallicum*, it is prescribed for cramps and whooping cough. Chinese physicians use copper as a painkiller and decongestant to relieve the pain and swelling of bruises, fractures, and dislocations.

PREPARATIONS: Injections, tablets, powder, homeopathic remedies, bracelet.

CAUTION: **Excess copper is toxic.**

Cynara scolymus (Compositae)
GLOBE ARTICHOKE

A popular vegetable since Greek and Roman times, it is now a scientifically-proven liver remedy; it promotes the healing of liver tissue and can reduce blood cholesterol levels. A native of North Africa but widely cultivated around the world, the plant is a tall perennial with very long, divided leaves that are greenish gray on top and whitish beneath. Purple flowers appear in late summer and are large and thistlelike, with soft spikes.

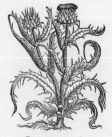

***Cynara* species**

PARTS USED: Flower head, leaves, root.

ACTIVE INGREDIENTS: Cynarin; sesquiterpene lactones; alkaloids; flavonoids, including scolymoside; inulin; tannins.

ACTIONS: Increases the flow of bile; heals liver cells; increases urine production; bitter (digestive stimulant).

MEDICINAL USE: Given for gallbladder and bile diseases, and liver damage caused by toxins, alcohol, or hepatitis. It is also prescribed for raised blood cholesterol levels, and kidney diseases that result in protein in the urine.

PREPARATIONS: Juice, infusion, vegetable, tincture.

Cypripedium calceolus var. *pubescens* (Orchidaceae)
LARGE YELLOW LADY'S SLIPPER, AMERICAN VALERIAN, NERVEROOT

A remedy passed on to the white settlers by Native Americans, it is a native of the eastern United States and first appeared in Europe during the 18th century. It is such an effective sedative that it was called American valerian after the European valerian renowned for its sedative properties. One of the few orchids used in medicine, it has a fleshy root and pointed leaves on soft, glandular, hairy stems. Bright yellow flowers appear in late summer. It is found in boggy, rich soils, but is an endangered species and should not be collected in the wild.

PARTS USED: Root.

ACTIVE INGREDIENTS: Volatile oil; glycosides; resins; tannins.

ACTIONS: Sedative; mildly promotes sleep; reduces muscle tension and spasms.

MEDICINAL USE: Used in insomnia, hysteria, nervous tension, and anxiety. It is also particularly helpful as an aid to recovery from chronic conditions. Other species of orchid are prescribed in Chinese medicine for fevers, restlessness, and thirst.

PREPARATIONS: Decoction, infusion, tincture

Datura stramonium (Solanaceae)
JIMSONWEED, COMMON THORN APPLE, DEVIL'S APPLE, JAMESTOWN WEED

The unpleasant effects that datura produces if misused, such as double vision and hallucinations, led to its common name of devil's apple. Despite these effects, the herbalist Gerard recommended a salve made from the leaves for "all inflammations whatsoever." The origins of this widely naturalized plant are unclear, but it is claimed to be a native of both western Asia and South America. It was introduced to Europe as a drug in the 16th century, and is a strong-smelling annual with large, soft, oval leaves. Funnel-shaped, bluish white flowers appear in late summer and are followed by an egg-shaped capsule covered in spines, which opens into four segments containing the brown seeds.

PARTS USED: Leaves, seeds.

ACTIVE INGREDIENTS: Tropane alkaloids, including hyoscamine, hyoscine, and atropine.

ACTIONS: Reduces muscle tension and spasms; relieves asthma; blocks a part of the nervous system (cholinergic) to prevent muscle contractions.

MEDICINAL USE: Given for the relief of bronchial spasms in asthma and the muscle spasms associated with Parkinson's disease. It is used for similar purposes in Ayurvedic medicine.

PREPARATIONS: Infusion, tincture, smoked leaf.

CAUTION: **Poisonous, use only on the advice of a qualified practitioner.**

Daucus carota (Umbelliferae)
WILD CARROT, QUEEN ANNE'S LACE

Known since Greek and Roman times as a medicinal herb and vegetable, it is native to Europe, North Africa, and western Asia but the fleshier domestic form is now cultivated throughout the world. It is a biennial with finely divided leaves and a hard, thin, whitish root that has a disagreeable taste. In early to midsummer, clusters of small, white flowers with a few purple or red ones in the center appear and then develop into dry, flattened fruit.

PARTS USED: Whole herb, seeds.

ACTIVE INGREDIENTS: Volatile oil in the seeds, including pinene, carotol, daucol, limonene, and gerianol; alkaloid, daucine; in the root, vitamin C and carotene.

ACTIONS: Increases urine production; prevents the formation of kidney stones; relieves gas and colic.

MEDICINAL USE: Given to prevent the formation of urinary stones, and to treat cystitis and gout. The seeds are useful for colic and flatulence and are also used to promote menstruation. The herb has similar uses in Ayurvedic medicine.

PREPARATIONS: Infusion, tincture, seeds.

Demospongiae ✹
HORNY SPONGE

This living sponge looks like a slimy piece of raw liver. Different kinds of horny sponge exist throughout the warm seas of the world, but they have been so overfished in the Mediterranean that their survival there is threatened. All horny sponges contain an elastic substance known as hornin, which is chemically related to silk and horn.

PARTS USED: Burnt whole sponge.

ACTIVE INGREDIENTS: Iodine.

ACTIONS: Stops bleeding from external wounds; astringent; anti-inflammatory.

MEDICINAL USE: In Unani medicine, it is applied externally to swollen glands and to eyes to improve eyesight, and is also used for washing wounds and cavities. *Spongia tosta* (roasted sponge) is a homeopathic remedy for swollen thyroid glands, headaches, and coughs.

PREPARATIONS: Sponge ash mixed in oil or made into a surma (paste), homeopathic remedies.

Digitalis purpurea & D. lanata
(Scrophulariaceae) ✹☠
FOXGLOVE

Until the late 18th century, European herbalists used the leaves of digitalis purely for the healing of wounds and skin diseases. It was only when an English doctor, William Withering, discovered that foxglove was the active herb in a folk recipe for dropsy that its value in the treatment of heart disease was recognized. Today, glycosides are extracted from *D. purpurea* and *D. lanata* by the pharmaceutical industry to produce the heart drugs digitoxin and digoxin respectively. Native to western Europe, the plants are biennial with a rosette of downy, oval leaves, from which rises a spike of purple (*D. purpurea*) or white (*D. lanata*) trumpetlike flowers in midsummer.

PARTS USED: Leaves.

ACTIVE INGREDIENTS: Cardioactive glycosides, including purpurea glycosides A and B, giving rise to digitoxin and gitoxin in *D. purpurea*, and lanatosides A, B, and C, giving rise to digitoxin, gitoxin, and digoxin in *D. lanata*.

ACTIONS: Increases the efficiency of the heartbeat; increases urine production.

MEDICINAL USE: Prescribed throughout the world for heart failure and to regulate heartbeat, only the extracted pharmaceutical drugs are used in the United States and Canada, although the leaf has been shown to be less toxic and to be required in smaller doses.

PREPARATIONS: Leaf extract, pharmaceutical preparations.

CAUTION: **Use only under the guidance of a qualified practitioner.**

Dioscorea villosa (Dioscoriaceae) ✹
WILD YAM, COLIC ROOT, RHEUMATISM ROOT

A native of eastern and central United States, yam grows widely throughout the tropics, where it is used as a starchy root crop. Until 1970, a related species of wild yam, *D. mexicana*, was the sole source of sex hormones for the manufacture of the female contraceptive pill. Today, many species of *Dioscorea*, including wild yam, are used in the preparation of steroids by the pharmaceutical industry. Wild yam is a perennial with long, twisted roots, a twining stem, small heart-shaped leaves, and green to yellow flowers that appear in summer.

PARTS USED: Root or rhizome.

ACTIVE INGREDIENTS: Steroidal saponins based on diosgenin, including dioscin and dioscorin; starch; tannins.

ACTIONS: Reduces muscle tension and spasms; dilates local blood vessels; increases the flow of bile; anti-inflammatory.

MEDICINAL USE: Used in the treatment of rheumatic diseases. Also given for colic, inflammation of the colon, cramps, intermittent claudication (pain in the calves caused by spasms in the blood vessels supplying the leg muscles), menstrual cramps, and ovarian and uterine pain. Related species are commonly prescribed in Chinese medicine for dysentery, indigestion, asthma, and rheumatoid arthritis, and in Ayurvedic medicine for impotence, infertility, abdominal cramps, and hysteria. Homeopathically, *Dioscorea* is given for stomach pain.

PREPARATIONS: Decoction, tincture, pharmaceutical preparations, homeopathic remedies.

Dolomite ⬡
CALCIUM MAGNESIUM CARBONATE

Named after D. Dolomieu, the French geologist who identified it, dolomite is one of the most common mountain rocks. This is a remarkable fact considering it originates from the shells of tiny sea animals that have been deposited in the sea and, over millions of years, turned into translucent, colorless, white, or pink crystals.

PARTS USED: Whole mineral.

ACTIVE INGREDIENTS: Calcium; magnesium.

ACTIONS: Nutrient.

MEDICINAL USE: Dolomite is used to supplement calcium and magnesium deficiencies, caused, for instance, by reliance on refined food, heavy alcohol consumption, or long-term drug therapy. The symptoms of deficiency that it is used for include muscular weakness and cramps.

PREPARATIONS: Tablets.

Drosera rotundifolia (Droseraceae) ✹
ROUND-LEAVED SUNDEW

This small plant is insectivorous, catching its prey on the sticky secretions produced by glandular hairs on its leaves. Found throughout the world in damp, acid, boggy places, it is a perennial with orb-shaped

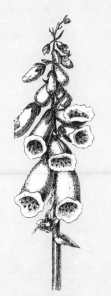

Digitalis purpurea

leaves and a complete covering of red hairs. Small white flowers appear throughout the summer and autumn.

PARTS USED: Whole herb.
ACTIVE INGREDIENTS: Napthaquinones, including plumbagin; flavonoids.
ACTIONS: Expectorant; reduces muscle tension and spasms; antimicrobial.
MEDICINAL USE: Given to relieve bronchial spasms in asthmatics, whooping cough, and bronchitis, and also for stomach ulcers. Used in homeopathy (*Drosera*) for coughs and sore throats. Chinese physicians prescribe *Drosera* species for dysentery, headaches, and rheumatic pains.
PREPARATIONS: Infusion, tincture, homeopathic remedies.

Echinacea angustifolia (Compositae) 🌿
PURPLE CONEFLOWER, KANSAS SNAKEROOT

For over 100 years, the coneflower has been known to increase resistance to infections; both Native Americans and the early settlers used it to clean and heal wounds, against infectious disease, and even to cure snakebites. Scientific research has now confirmed its stimulatory effects on the white blood cells that fight infection, and it is being studied in California as a possible treatment for AIDS. A native of central and southwestern United States and widely grown in gardens across the world, it is a perennial with coarse, hairy stems and leaves. Flowers comprising a central, raised, daisylike cone and an outer ring of purple florets, appear in late summer.

PARTS USED: Root, rhizome.
ACTIVE INGREDIENTS: Phenylcarbonic acid glycosides, including echinacoside and echinacin; volatile oil containing humulene and caryophyllene; flavonoids; polysaccharides; polyacetylenes.
ACTIONS: Antiseptic; antiviral; stimulates the immune system; stimulates nutrition and elimination processes to greater efficiency.
MEDICINAL USE: Prescribed as an aid for wound healing, particularly for boils and carbuncles, and to treat septicemia (blood poisoning) and upper respiratory tract infections, including influenza, tonsilitis, and pharyngitis.
PREPARATIONS: Decoction, tincture.

Elettaria cardamomum (Zingiberaceae) 🌿
CARDAMOM, ILACHI, MALABAR CARDAMOM

Cardamom fruits have long been used as a spice in curry powder and by the Egyptians to flavor coffee. The seeds were known to Dioscorides in 77 AD and are mentioned in the *Arabian Nights*. A relative of ginger, cardamom is native to the wet tropical hills of southern India. Cardamom is a perennial with a thick root and large, oval, pointed leaves. Its flowers are small and yellow with a purple lip and its seeds are encased in a thin, papery pod to form the well-known cardamom fruit.

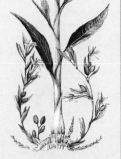

Elettaria cardamomum

PARTS USED: Seeds.
ACTIVE INGREDIENTS: Volatile oil with cineole, limonene, terpineol, and linalool.
ACTIONS: Relieves gas and colic; increases the flow of saliva; stimulates the appetite.
MEDICINAL USE: Given for flatulent indigestion and to stimulate the appetite in people with anorexia. It is prescribed in Ayurvedic medicine for coughs, colds, bronchitis, asthma, and indigestion, and Chinese medicine uses it as a tonic and for urinary incontinence.
PREPARATIONS: Seeds, infusion, tincture.

Ephedra sinica (Ephedraceae) 🌿
MA HUANG

Ephedra has been used as a treatment for asthma in Chinese medicine for 5,000 years. However, it was not until 1887 that the drug ephedrine was isolated from the plant, which is still used as a source of ephedrine and pseudoephedrine by the pharmaceutical industry. Ephedrine alone is used less commonly for asthma today because it may raise blood pressure dangerously. However, the whole plant is safer, as it contains other ingredients that help to lower blood pressure while ephedrine eases the asthma. Native to the Himalayas and China, it is a short shrub with smooth, green, grooved branches and leaves reduced to tufts. Its flowers are produced in summer and are followed by small, succulent cones.

PARTS USED: Young stems.
ACTIVE INGREDIENTS: Alkaloids, including ephedrine pseudoephedrine, and norephedrine.
ACTIONS: Relieves asthma; dilates the lung passages; stimulates the heart; constricts local blood vessels.
MEDICINAL USE: Given for asthma to relieve the severity and frequency of spasms of the lung passages, and for hives, hay fever, and other allergies. Chinese physicians also prescribe it for colds, influenza, coughs, joint pain, and swelling. Ephedrine and pseudoephedrine are ingredients in several pharmaceutical preparations for the relief of coughs and colds.
PREPARATIONS: Infusion, tincture, pharmaceutical preparations.
CAUTION: Only use under the guidance of a qualified practitioner. All products containing ephedrine or pseuodephedrine should be avoided by people with high blood pressure, glaucoma, and hyperthyroidism or in patients taking MAOI (monoamine oxidase inhibitor) antidepressant drugs.

Epsomite 🪨
EPSOM SALTS, HYDRATED MAGNESIUM SULFATE

Named after a spring in Epsom, Surrey, which contains the mineral magnesium sulfate in solution, Epsom salts have enjoyed a huge usage that some people think is undeserved. Magnesium sulfate can still be found in many remedies for constipation and overindulgence.

PARTS USED: Whole mineral.
ACTIVE INGREDIENTS: Magnesium sulfate.
ACTIONS: Laxative.
MEDICINAL USE: Used in orthodox medicine for constipation and hangovers, and as a supplement for magnesium deficiency.
PREPARATIONS: Salt, tablets, and liquid mixtures are available over the counter, but should be used with caution.

Equisetum arvense (Equisetaceae)
HORSETAIL, BOTTLEBRUSH, SHAVE GRASS

This ancient plant, which is a common fossil in coal deposits, has been used since Roman times as a vegetable, an animal feed, and a medicine. Culpeper said it was "very powerful to stop bleeding, either inward or outward and eases the swelling, heat, and inflammation of the fundamental, or privy parts, in men and women." Native to Europe, it has two types of stem that grow from a wandering rhizome – fertile stems in early spring, followed by vegetative stems.

PARTS USED: Vegetative stems.
ACTIVE INGREDIENTS: Alkaloids, including nicotine, palustrine, and palustrinine; saponins; flavonoids, including isoquercitrin and equicetrin; sterols, including cholesterol; silicic acid; minerals.
ACTIONS: Halts or reduces bleeding (external and internal); astringent; stimulates immune response.
MEDICINAL USE: Given for urinary and prostate diseases to relieve symptoms and aid healing, for bed-wetting, and for lung damage caused by TB and other lung disease. *E. hiemale* is prescribed by Chinese doctors for eye disorders, dysentery, flu, swelling, and hemorrhoids.
PREPARATIONS: Infusion, tincture.

Eruca sativa (Cruciferae)
ROCKET, ROCQUETTE, ROCKET-SALAD

Rocket has been a salad vegetable and medicine in southern Europe since Roman times and is now popular in France, Italy, and Egypt. In the past, it was associated with deceit because the flower has a sweet perfume at night but none in the day. A native of Italy, it is an annual with a rosette of long, broadly-toothed, peppery-tasting leaves at its base, cream flowers with purple veins in summer, and pods containing mustardlike seeds in the autumn.

PARTS USED: Leaves.
ACTIVE INGREDIENTS: Volatile oil; heterosides.
ACTIONS: Prevents scurvy; stimulates digestion.
MEDICINAL USE: Used for digestive problems, support in lymphatic conditions, and scrofula (tuberculosis of bones or the lymphatic system).
PREPARATIONS: Fresh leaves.

Erythroxylum coca (Erythroxylaceae)
COCA, COCAINE PLANT

Peruvian Indians chew coca leaves to relieve hunger and fatigue, and it was this practice that led to the idea of basing Coca-Cola's original recipe on coca extracts. In 1902, however, use of the plant in the drink was banned because of its dangerous side effects. The first records of coca use date from 500 AD, but it was not until 1860 that the drug cocaine was first extracted. It is native to Peru and Bolivia but has been introduced to Indonesia. A shrubby tree with thick, oval leaves, it flowers in summer and produces small, round berries similar to coffee fruit.

PARTS USED: Leaves.
ACTIVE INGREDIENTS: Tropane alkaloids, including cocaine and cinnamyl-cocaine; glycosides; cocatannic acid; volatile oil containing methyl salicylate; flavonoids.
ACTIONS: Central nervous system stimulant; local anesthetic.
MEDICINAL USE: Its medicinal use is almost entirely restricted to that of a local anesthetic for minor surgical procedures. Occasionally, a mixture of morphine and cocaine (a Brompton cocktail) is prescribed for terminally ill patients to relieve pain and suffering.
PREPARATIONS: Leaf, tincture, pharmaceutical preparations.
CAUTION: **A restricted drug in most countries; possession is illegal.**

Eucalyptus globulus (Myrtaceae)
BLUE GUM, TASMANIAN BLUE GUM

Eucalyptus, or gum, trees are the most characteristic feature of the Australian flora. Yorkshireman and Australian emigrant Joseph Bosito first discovered the volatile oils in eucalyptus in 1848, and began distilling them. Commercial production started in Victoria in 1860 and, since then, out of the 300 species discovered, 30 have found medicinal use. The tree's amazing ability to dry out marshy soil also led to its use in eradicating the malaria mosquito in Africa, southern Europe, and India. Eucalyptus grows to 375 feet and has a smooth blue-gray trunk, and long, narrow, leathery leaves with a bluish green hue and many oil glands. Flowering during late summer, it also produces fruit shaped like spinning tops and coated with powdery wax.

PARTS USED: Oil from leaves.
ACTIVE INGREDIENTS: Volatile oil containing mainly 1,8-cineole (eucalyptol), terpineole, and pinene; polyphenolic acids, including caffeic and gallic; flavonoids, including eucalyptin, hyperoside, and rutin.
ACTIONS: Antiseptic; reduces muscle tension and spasms; expectorant; stimulant; reduces or prevents fever.
MEDICINAL USE: Used as an ingredient of cough mixtures and other pharmaceutical preparations. It is also given as an inhalant and applied externally as a vapor rub for colds, other chest infections, and bruised or strained muscles.
PREPARATIONS: Essential oil, tincture, rub, pharmaceutical preparations.

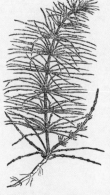
Equisetum arvense

Eupatorium perfoliatum (Compositae) ✦
BONESET, FEVERWORT, THOROUGHWORT

This North American herb was a boon to the early white settlers, who used it to treat a serious flulike disease called break bone fever. This led to the name boneset, while Native Americans called it ague weed. Native to the East Coast of North America and growing in marshy soils, it is a perennial with spear-shaped leaves and small white or bluish flowers in late summer.

PARTS USED: Whole herb.
ACTIVE INGREDIENTS: Volatile oil, containing sesquiterpene lactones; glycoside, eupatorin; polysaccharides; flavonoids, including quercitin, kaempferol, and rutin.
ACTIONS: Dilates peripheral (local) blood vessels; induces sweating; increases the flow of bile; reduces muscle tension and spasms; mild laxative.
MEDICINAL USE: Particularly used for flu associated with muscle pain. It is also given for bronchitis, persistent nasal catarrh, and rheumatic conditions made worse by dampness. Chinese medicine uses it for summer colds, heatstroke, tightness of the chest, and bad breath. In homeopathy, *Eupatorium* is prescribed for flu and malaria.
PREPARATIONS: Infusion, tincture, homeopathic remedies.

Euphorbia hirta (Euphorbiaceae) ✦
PILL-BEARING SPURGE, ASTHMA WEED

Pill-bearing spurge is one of the few safe medicinal plants among the several thousand species in its family. Most Euphorbiaceae contain a milky latex that can be very poisonous, for example, *E. heptagona* is used in poisoned arrows in East Africa. Native to India but naturalized throughout the tropics, *E. hirta* grows freely on waste ground and roadsides, and as a garden weed. It can be annual or perennial and has low, spreading stems and oval leaves, both of which are reddish and hairy. Tight clusters of small flowers appear in summer, followed by capsules containing tiny red seeds.

PARTS USED: Whole herb.
ACTIVE INGREDIENTS: Flavonoids, including quercetin; terpenoids; phenolic acids; choline.
ACTIONS: Antiasthmatic; expectorant; reduces muscle tension and spasms; kills and helps expel worms; kills amoebae.
MEDICINAL USE: Given for asthma, bronchitis, and upper respiratory catarrh. Used against amebic dysentery in the tropics. Chinese physicians prescribe it for athlete's foot and other skin conditions, as well as dysentery.
PREPARATIONS: Infusion, tincture.

Euphrasia officinalis (Scrophulariaceae) ✦
EYEBRIGHT, EUPHRASY, CASSE LUNETTE

Although this herb is named after Euphrosyne, one of the three Greek Graces, there are no records of its medicinal use by the ancient Greeks. First records of such use are from the 14th century when the herbalist Hildegarde recommended it to "strengthen the head, eyes, and memory." A native of Europe but found in western Asia and North America, it is a semiparasitic plant, always growing in association with meadow grass. Eyebright is an annual with oval, toothed leaves and, in mid- to late summer, flowers that have a double-lobed lower lip with a yellow patch and fine red or purple veins resembling a bloodshot eye.

PARTS USED: Whole herb.
ACTIVE INGREDIENTS: Iridoid glycosides, including acubin; tannins; phenolic acids; volatile oil; choline.
ACTIONS: Relieves catarrh; astringent; anti-inflammatory.
MEDICINAL USE: Given as an astringent for nasal and upper respiratory catarrh, sinusitis, and conjunctivitis. It is also used in homeopathy (*Euphrasia*) for hay fever.
PREPARATIONS: Infusion, tincture, extract, homeopathic remedies.

Fagopyrum esculentum (Polygonaceae) ✦
BUCKWHEAT, BLÉ NOIR, SARACEN CORN

Buckwheat is not related to bread wheat but is used as a flour in central Asia and China, where it is native, as a grain in Russia, and to make pancakes in North America. An annual with erect stems, soft arrow-shaped leaves, and small, pinkish flowers in summer, it also produces small seeds shaped like three-sided pyramids.

PARTS USED: Leaves.
ACTIVE INGREDIENTS: Flavonoid glycosides, rutin, and quercetin.
ACTIONS: Prevents hemorrhage; dilates the blood vessels; repairs blood vessel walls.
MEDICINAL USE: Used to treat high blood pressure associated with fragile capillaries, and for frostbite, chilblains (sores caused by exposure to extreme cold), retinal hemorrhages, and radiation damage. In Chinese medicine, it is prescribed for traumatic injuries, lumbago, menstrual cramps, bites, and stings.
PREPARATIONS: Infusion, tablets.

Ferula assa-foetida (Umbelliferae) ✦
ASAFETIDA, DEVIL'S DUNG,
FOOD OF THE GODS

The fetid, unpleasant smell of this plant is acknowledged in its Latin name and in the common name devil's dung. It was used medicinally in Arabia in the 2nd century, and was recorded by the Welsh physicians of Myddvai around the 13th century. Indian cooks use it as a condiment with "windy vegetables," and it is contained in the secret spice mix of the famous Worcestershire sauce. Asafetida is native to Afghanistan and Iran, where it grows up to 4,000 feet above sea level. A tall perennial, it has large fernlike leaves, a thick rootstock, and flowers in the spring of its fifth year.

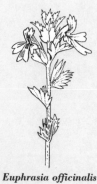

Euphrasia officinalis

PARTS USED: Oleo-gum resin from the root.
ACTIVE INGREDIENTS: Resin; gum; volatile oil; ferulic acid; coumarins.
ACTIONS: Reduces muscle tension and spasms; relieves gas and colic; expectorant.
MEDICINAL USE: Given for indigestion, flatulence, colic, nervous irritability (particularly in children), and bronchitis. In Ayurvedic medicine, it is prescribed for similar purposes, as well as for whooping cough, epilepsy, asthma, paralysis, and worms.
PREPARATIONS: Powdered resin, tablets.

Ficaria ranunculoides/Ranunculus ficaria (Ranunculaceae) 🖉
PILEWORT, SMALL CELANDINE, FIGWORT

Pilewort's Latin name comes from *rana*, meaning frog, because plants of this species grow in damp and waterlogged places. It is a classic example of the ancient "doctrine of signatures" (using plants medicinally for conditions they resemble). Pilewort has small, fat tubers that look like hemorrhoids and it has been used for hemorrhoids since the Middle Ages. Native to Europe and western Asia, it is one of the first spring flowers. A perennial with creeping stems and dark green, heart-shaped leaves, it has yellow flowers that open in bright sunlight.

PARTS USED: Whole herb.
ACTIVE INGREDIENTS: Saponins; protoanaemonin and anemonin; tannins.
ACTIONS: Astringent; constricts blood vessels.
MEDICINAL USE: Used both externally and internally for hemorrhoids.
PREPARATIONS: Cream, suppositories, tablets.

Filipendula ulmaria/Spiraea ulmaria (Rosaceae) 🖉
MEADOWSWEET, QUEEN OF THE MEADOW

Meadowsweet was one of the plants from which salicylic acid, the aspirinlike painkiller, was extracted. Using the whole plant, however, is safer than using the extracted drug, as it does not cause stomach bleeding, which is common with aspirin and related drugs. Native to Europe and Asia but now naturalized in North America, it is a perennial with reddish stems, serrated leaflets, and tiny, white or cream, sweet-scented flowers in mid- to late summer.

PARTS USED: Whole herb.
ACTIVE INGREDIENTS: Salicylic glycosides, including spiraein and gaultherin; flavonoids, including rutin, spiraeoside, and hyperoside; tannins; coumarin; ascorbic acid.
ACTIONS: Stimulates the stomach; antirheumatic; neutralizes excess stomach acid; induces sweating; anti-inflammatory; astringent; urinary antiseptic.
MEDICINAL USE: Used for peptic ulceration and other damage to the lining of the stomach associated with excess acid, such as indigestion and heartburn. It is also given for rheumatic pain, and for diarrhea in children.
PREPARATIONS: Infusion, tincture.

Fluorite 🖾
CALCIUM FLUORIDE, FLUORSPAR

Occurring naturally as beautiful crystals in a rainbow of colors, fluorite is the main source of fluorine, an element that is highly poisonous yet an essential trace mineral. We obtain much of this essential fluorine as sodium fluoride from water. However, the amount of this salt in water varies widely from area to area. In low sodium fluoride areas, tooth decay is high and in very high areas, irreversible tooth mottling is common, hence the controversy about how much we should depend on the addition of sodium fluoride to our water supply to prevent tooth decay. Fluoridated toothpastes and tooth paints provide a way of benefiting from fluoride without the risks associated with swallowing it.

PARTS USED: Fluorite in its natural state or to make sodium fluoride.
ACTIVE INGREDIENTS: Fluorine; calcium fluoride.
ACTIONS: Nutrient; prevents tooth decay.
MEDICINAL USE: Given to make teeth more resistant to decay. Chinese medicine recommends fluorite for insomnia and anxiety, for coughs and wheezing, and for excessive bleeding from the uterus. The homeopathic remedy *Calcarea fluorata* is used for hemorrhoids, varicose veins, boils, and arthritis, and to prevent tooth decay.
PREPARATIONS: Drops, tooth paint, toothpaste, decoctions, homeopathic remedies.

Foeniculum vulgare (Umbelliferae) 🖉
FENNEL, FENKEL

The fine, hairlike leaves of this plant led the Romans to call it *Foeniculum*, meaning little hay. Highly respected as both a food and a medicine in ancient Rome and Greece, it was thought to have magical powers in medieval times and was hung over doors to keep out witches. Native to southern Europe, it is now naturalized all over the world and is widely cultivated for medicinal use. It is a hardy perennial with a blue-green, ribbed stem, feathery leaves, and umbrellalike clusters of yellow flowers in mid- to late summer, followed by grayish, oblong fruit that taste of anise.

PARTS USED: Fruit.
ACTIVE INGREDIENTS: Volatile oil containing anethole, fenchone, limonene, and apiole; flavonoids, including rutin, kaempferol, and quercetin; coumarins, including bergapten.
ACTIONS: Stimulates the stomach; relieves gas and colic; anti-inflammatory; stimulates the appetite; stimulates milk production.
MEDICINAL USE: Given for indigestion associated with flatulence and colic (particularly in children), inflammation of the eyes or mouth, and to stimulate milk production in women who are breast-feeding. Chinese medicine prescribes fennel for food poisoning, hernias, abdominal pain, and indigestion.
PREPARATIONS: Infusion, dried fruit, tincture.

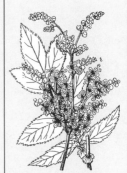

Filipendula ulmaria/ Spiraea ulmaria

Fucus vesiculosus (Fucaceae)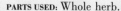
BLADDERWRACK, BLACK-TANG, CUTWEED, ROCKWEED

Farmers in the south of England use bladderwrack as a potash fertilizer, and it has long been used as an anti-òbesity medicine, probably because it has a high iodine content and may stimulate the thyroid gland, which controls the body's metabolic rate. Iodine is filtered out of seawater and stored by many seaweeds, which were a major source of iodine in the 19th century. Native to the North Atlantic and found along European and North American coastlines, this perennial algae has a flat, brown to olive-brown, fanlike thallus, or frond, with opposite pairs of air sacs, and is rooted to rocks near the low water mark.

PARTS USED: Thallus.
ACTIVE INGREDIENTS: Phenolic compounds; mucopolysaccharides, including algin; inorganic salts of iodine, bromine, and potassium.
ACTIONS: Stimulates the thyroid gland; anti-obesity; antirheumatic.
MEDICINAL USE: Used internally to treat obesity associated with an underactive thyroid gland and externally for rheumatic pains.
PREPARATIONS: Dried thallus, tincture, tablets.

Galipea officinalis (Rutaceae) *
ANGOSTURA, CUSPARIA BARK

Angostura was used for centuries by Native South Americans as a bitter tonic, and also as an aid to fishing because it stunned fish when added to the water. It was introduced to Europe in 1759, when it became an ingredient of the famous drink angostura bitters. Recently, however, it has been replaced in the drink by *Gentiana lutea*. Native to the mountains of South America, it is a perennial tree with three-lobed, glossy green leaves and nauseous-smelling flowers.

PARTS USED: Dried bark.
ACTIVE INGREDIENTS: Bitter principles; alkaloids, including cusparine and galipine; volatile oil.
ACTIONS: Aromatic bitter; tonic; stimulant; causes vomiting in large doses.
MEDICINAL USE: Used for digestive problems such as diarrhea, dysentery, and indigestion.
PREPARATIONS: Infusion, tincture, tablets.

Galium aparine (Rubiaceae) *
CLEAVERS, BEDSTRAW, GOOSEGRASS

A centuries-old treatment for skin diseases and blood purification, cleavers is still a popular "spring cleansing" tonic. Culpeper recommended it as a good remedy "to cleanse the blood and strengthen the liver, thereby to keep the body in health, and fitting it for that change of season that is coming." It is native to Europe, where it grows in moist waste places. A trailing annual, it has leaves and stems covered in fine hooks that cling to anything they touch.

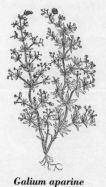

Galium aparine

PARTS USED: Whole herb.
ACTIVE INGREDIENTS: Iridoid coumarins, including asperuloside; flavonoids; tannins.
ACTIONS: Increases urine production; astringent; stimulates lymphatic drainage.
MEDICINAL USE: Given for eczema-type skin eruptions, swollen lymph glands (particularly if associated with water retention), urinary infections, and kidney stones.
PREPARATIONS: Infusion, tincture.

Gaultheria procumbens (Ericaceae) *
WINTERGREEN, TEABERRY, CHECKERBERRY

Wintergreen used to be a major source of natural methyl salicylates (anti-inflammatory drugs), but most of the wintergreen oil containing methyl salicylates sold today is synthetic. A native of North America, it thrives on poor, dry, and sandy soils. It is a small, perennial, shrubby plant with stiff, erect branches, tufts of oval leaves, and drooping white flowers that appear in midsummer and develop into red berries.

PARTS USED: Leaves.
ACTIVE INGREDIENTS: Volatile oil containing methyl salicylate; phenolic compounds, including salicylic, gaultherin, vanillic, and caffeic acids.
ACTIONS: Anti-inflammatory; increases urine production; antirheumatic.
MEDICINAL USE: Applied externally to relieve the pain of rheumatism, myalgia (muscle pain), sprains, and sciatica. Methyl salicylate is an ingredient of several pharmaceutical preparations.
PREPARATIONS: Ointment, liniment, cream.

Gelsemium sempervirens (Loganiaceae) *☠
YELLOW JESSAMINE, FALSE JASMINE, EVENING TRUMPET FLOWER

Yellow jessamine was originally used for fevers by early North American settlers, but has come to be used mainly for facial neuralgia (nerve pain). A native of North America, it is poisonous and is in no way related to the scented European jasmines. Growing near water in rich, damp, lowland soils, this perennial climber has spear-shaped leaves and clusters of fragrant, trumpet-shaped, yellow flowers in early spring.

PARTS USED: Roots and rhizome.
ACTIVE INGREDIENTS: Alkaloids, including gelsemine, gelsemedine, and gelsedine; iridoids, including gelsemide; coumarins; tannins.
ACTIONS: Sedative; relieves pain; induces sweating; reduces muscle tension and spasms.
MEDICINAL USE: Used externally for facial neuralgia and toothache. The homeopathic remedy (*Gelsemium*) is given for dull headaches associated with fever, colds and catarrh, sore throats, tonsillitis, and flu.
PREPARATIONS: Tincture, homeopathic remedies.
CAUTION: **Highly poisonous. Sale of the herb is restricted in the U.S. and Canada, and it should be used only under the guidance of a qualified practitioner.**

Gentiana lutea (Gentianaceae) 🌢
YELLOW GENTIAN

Gentian is an ancient medicine whose name is said to have come from Gentius, King of Illyria, who discovered its ability to neutralize poisons. Containing one of the most bitter substances known to man, gentian is used as a scientific reference for bitterness. An alpine plant found at about 4,000 feet above sea level, it is native to Europe and Asia Minor but is distributed widely around the world. The root, which is thick and long, throws up an erect stem with short, stalkless, yellowish leaves. Yellow flowers appear in spring.

PARTS USED: Dried root.
ACTIVE INGREDIENTS: Bitter seco-iridoid glycosides, including gentiopicroside, gentioside, amarogentin, and swertismarin; xanthones, including gentisein and gentisin; alkaloids, including gentianine; phenolic acids.
ACTIONS: Strong bitter stimulant; anti-inflammatory.
MEDICINAL USE: Used to treat sluggish digestion, anorexia, inflammation of the digestive tract such as indigestion, and liver and gallbladder diseases such as hepatitis. Other species of *Gentiana* are prescribed in Chinese medicine for similar conditions, as well as for conjunctivitis, urinary tract infections, eczema, and other skin problems. Some over-the-counter tonic preparations still contain gentian.
PREPARATIONS: Dried root, tincture, tablets.

Geranium maculatum (Gerianaceae) 🌢
WILD GERANIUM, ALUMROOT, SPOTTED CRANESBILL

The generic name of this species is derived from the Greek for crane, because the unripe fruit looks like a crane's bill. It was a favorite herb of Native Americans, who used it as an astringent. Native to North America, it is a perennial with a hairy stem and lobed, pale green leaves that become spotted with age. Rose-pink flowers appear in late summer.

PARTS USED: Rhizome.
ACTIVE INGREDIENTS: Tannins, including gallic acid.
ACTIONS: Astringent; stops bleeding from external wounds; promotes wound healing; tonic.
MEDICINAL USE: Given internally to control diarrhea, food poisoning, peptic ulcers, and inflammatory bowel disease. Used locally as a mouthwash for mouth infections and ulcers, and as a douche for vaginal infections.
PREPARATIONS: Dried rhizome, tincture, tablets.

Glechoma hederacea/Nepeta hederacea (Labiatae) 🌢
GROUND IVY, CAT'S PAW

Ground ivy has long been used as a cure for coughs and consumption, especially by the impoverished, who were more prone to such illnesses because of their inadequate housing and nutrition. Native to Europe but naturalized in North America and widely found in temperate regions on sunny waste ground and by hedgerows and banks, it is not related to true ivy (*Hedera* spp.) but resembles it. A low-growing perennial, it has square stems, dark green, heart-shaped leaves, and purple-pink flowers in spring.

PARTS USED: Whole herb.
ACTIVE INGREDIENTS: Sesquiterpenes; flavonoids, including quercetin, hyperoside, and apigenin; saponins; bitter principle, glechomine.
ACTIONS: Astringent; relieves catarrh; promotes wound healing; increases urine production.
MEDICINAL USE: Given to treat chronic catarrh, bronchitis, cystitis, and tinnitus (ringing in the ears). It is also used to help reduce the symptoms of mild diarrhea, hemorrhoids, and gastritis. The Chinese prescribe it for flu, kidney stones, trauma, rheumatoid arthritis, and skin sores.
PREPARATIONS: Dried herb, infusion, tincture.

Glycyrrhiza glabra (Leguminosae) 🌢
LICORICE, LACRISSE, SWEET ROOT

Licorice was one of the most widely known medicines in ancient history, and records of its use abound in manuscripts ranging from the Assyrian tablets of about 2,000 BC to Chinese herbals from the same period. Today, licorice extracts are used in pharmaceutical drugs for peptic ulcers, and as a general flavoring for drugs and foods. Native to Europe and Asia, licorice is widely grown around the world, and several species have been used for commercial extracts. A complex of thick roots sends up erect stems bearing leaves of oval leaflets and clusters of small pink to violet flowers during mid- to late summer.

PARTS USED: Root.
ACTIVE INGREDIENTS: Glycyrrhizin; glycyrrhetinic acid; flavonoids and isoflavonoids; coumarins.
ACTIONS: Stimulates the cortex of the adrenal gland; soothes internal body surfaces; anti-inflammatory; expectorant; reduces muscle tension and spasms; mimics estrogen; antiallergic; a liver protectant.
MEDICINAL USE: Given for peptic ulcers, which it both relieves and heals, bronchial catarrh, sore throats, gastritis (stomach inflammation), rheumatic conditions, and mild allergic asthma. One of the most widely used herbs in Chinese prescriptions, where it is given for abdominal pain, vomiting and diarrhea, chesty coughs, dry sore throats, abscesses, and hepatitis.
PREPARATIONS: Extract, tincture, tablets, pharmaceutical preparations.
CAUTION: **Long term usage at high doses may cause sodium retention, low potassium levels, and high blood pressure.**

Graphite 🞖
BLACK LEAD, PLUMBAGO

This dark gray form of carbon has been used in pencils since 1562, when the world's first pencil factory opened in Britain.

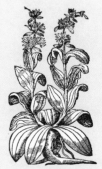

Gentiana lutea

However, it was not until the 19th century that graphite was given this name, after *graphein*, the Greek for to write. It has many other uses, from making lubricants to slowing down neutrons in nuclear reactors. In spite of its common names, graphite contains no lead.

PARTS USED: Whole mineral.
ACTIVE INGREDIENTS: Crystalline carbon.
ACTIONS: Soothes the skin.
MEDICINAL USE: A homeopathic remedy (*Graphites*) used for skin problems such as psoriasis, eczema, and cracked and weeping skin, and for hot flashes, amenorrhea, and premenstrual tension.
PREPARATIONS: Homeopathic remedies.

Gryllotalpa orientalis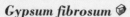
MOLE-CRICKET

Chinese enthusiasm for the cricket has produced an entire "cricket culture" based on cricket chirping competitions. Mole-crickets are an earth-tunnelling relative of the cricket; they have strong front legs for digging. Another of the mole-cricket's claims to fame is its strong smell.

PARTS USED: Bodies of males.
ACTIVE INGREDIENTS: Not known.
ACTIONS: Cooling; increases urine production.
MEDICINAL USE: Given in Chinese medicine for water retention, to ripen boils and abscesses to the bursting point, and for difficult labor.
PREPARATIONS: Roasted, powdered, and mixed with water.

Gypsum fibrosum
ALABASTER, CALCIUM SULFATE DIHYDRATE

Glassy or translucent, crystals of gypsum are found worldwide, occurring mostly as a result of evaporating seas and salt lakes. Burnt gypsum that has been ground into a white powder is known as plaster of Paris and is widely used to make plaster casts for broken bones, in cement for building, and as a fertilizer.

PARTS USED: Crystals.
ACTIVE INGREDIENTS: Calcium sulfate.
ACTIONS: Anti-inflammatory; helps reduce fever.
MEDICINAL USE: Prescribed internally by Chinese physicians for fevers and accompanying symptoms such as headaches, and also for coughs due to asthma and bronchitis, and externally for eczema, burns, and sores. Homeopathically, as *Calcarea sulphurea*, it is used for infections such as sinusitis with a yellow discharge.
PREPARATIONS: Powder, homeopathic remedies.

Haematitum
HEMATITE, NATIVE BROWN IRON OXIDE, IRON ORE

A common mineral and one of the main sources of iron since ancient times, hematite occurs naturally in crystals of iridescent charcoal gray, or mixed with red clay in kidneylike shapes.

Halite

PARTS USED: Clay version.
ACTIVE INGREDIENTS: Iron.
ACTIONS: Helps liver function; astringent; as a blood tonic; suppresses nausea and vomiting.
MEDICINAL USE: Chinese physicians use it for biliousness and symptoms such as dizziness, headaches, tinnitus (ringing in the ears), hiccups, nausea, and vomiting, and to stop bleeding.
PREPARATIONS: Powder.

Haliotis gigantea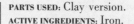
ABALONE, SEA EAR SHELLS

Ear-shaped abalone shells from the warm seas of the world are best known for their colorful pearly lining, which is often made into jewelry. The rather chewy clam contained within the shell is eaten. Abalone, which is a mollusk, clings to rocks with its muscular foot. The rows of holes in its shell are designed to enable it to breathe.

PARTS USED: Whole shell.
ACTIVE INGREDIENTS: Calcium carbonate; trace minerals.
ACTIONS: Sedative; helps reduce fever; lowers blood pressure.
MEDICINAL USE: Prescribed by Chinese physicians for a range of ailments, including fevers, headache, dizziness, red eyes, and blurred vision, particularly due to cataracts.
PREPARATIONS: Powdered shell or decoction internally; very fine powder externally on eyelids.

Halite
ROCK SALT, SODIUM CHLORIDE

In orthodox medicine, a high intake of salt is thought to increase the risk of high blood pressure, strokes, and heart disease. Homeopathically, however, sodium chloride is used for conditions ranging from colds to eczema. Both sodium and chloride are essential trace elements, but supplements are likely to be needed only after exceptional dehydration. Indeed, excess is more likely than deficiency, due to the large amount of salt added to common foods.

PARTS USED: Sodium chloride.
ACTIVE INGREDIENTS: Sodium chloride.
ACTIONS: Nutrient; preservative; absorbs water.
MEDICINAL USE: A homeopathic remedy (*Natrium muriaticum*) used for colds, sneezing, eczema, thrush, urticaria (hives), menstrual and premenstrual problems, and migraines. In Ayurvedic medicine, it is given to promote digestion, improve appetite, and relieve constipation. In orthodox medicine, sodium chloride solution is used for dehydration, to irrigate the eye, to relieve nasal congestion, and as a mouthwash.
PREPARATIONS: Homeopathic tablets, powder.

Hamamelis virginiana
(Hamamelidaceae)
WITCH HAZEL, SPOTTED ALDER

Witch hazel, now a common garden plant, was first employed by Native Americans, who used its twigs for water divining and its leaves and bark as a medicine for swellings and tumors. It has been widely used in pharmaceutical preparations for minor skin rashes and burns. Native to North America, it is a perennial shrub with a smooth bark, toothed, oval leaves, and yellow flowers that appear in very late summer, followed by small, black nuts containing white seeds.

PARTS USED: Leaves, bark.
ACTIVE INGREDIENTS: Tannins; flavonoids, including quercetin and kaempferol; saponins.
ACTIONS: Astringent; prevents hemorrhage; anti-inflammatory.
MEDICINAL USE: Applied externally for hemorrhoids, bruises, and inflamed swellings, and given internally for diarrhea and colitis (an inflammatory disease of the intestines). In homeopathy, *Hamamelis* is given for hemorrhoids and bleeding.
PREPARATIONS: Distilled extract, tincture, ointment, homeopathic remedies.

Harpagophylum procumbens
(Pedaliaceae) 🌶
DEVIL'S CLAW

One of the relatively small number of African plants included in European pharmacopoeias, devil's claw has powerful anti-inflammatory properties. These properties were confirmed in 1958, and medicinal use of the plant has since become widespread. It is native to South Africa and eastern Africa and grows in the desert. A perennial produced from large, globular tubers, it has violet or red trumpet-shaped flowers that develop into tough, barbed fruit which have been known to entangle and trap wild animals.

PARTS USED: Tuber.
ACTIVE INGREDIENTS: Iridoid glycosides, including harpagoside, harpagide, and procumbide; flavonoids, especially kaempferol and luteolin glycosides; phenolic acids.
ACTIONS: Anti-inflammatory; antirheumatic; relieves pain; sedative.
MEDICINAL USE: Particularly used to relieve the pain of rheumatism, arthritis, gout, myalgia (muscle pain), and lumbago (lower back pain).
PREPARATIONS: Powder, tincture.
CAUTION: **Avoid during pregnancy.**

Hippocampus kelloggi &
H. coronatus ⚥
SEA HORSE

The young of these beautiful fish are initially reared inside the male, who incubates eggs deposited there by the female. Different species occur in different parts of the world. Sea horse is a common ingredient in Chinese tonic mixtures.

PARTS USED: Whole.
ACTIVE INGREDIENTS: Not known.
ACTIONS: Tonic; stimulant.
MEDICINAL USE: A Chinese medicine used as a general tonic and for kidney problems, such as

difficulty in urinating. Chinese physicians also use alcoholic extractions for their hormone-stimulating effect.
PREPARATIONS: Powder, alcoholic extraction.

Hirudo medicinalis ⚥
LEECH

The widespread Western use of leeches to bleed patients as a remedy for almost any ailment only stopped some 100 years ago. As recently as 50 years ago, they were still used to treat black-and-blue spots on the skin, and live leeches are used in some hospitals today on certain patients who have undergone plastic surgery. Dead leeches continue to be used medically worldwide.

PARTS USED: Live, whole body, extracted enzymes.
ACTIVE INGREDIENTS: Hirudin; calin.
ACTIONS: Prevents blood clotting.
MEDICINAL USE: Live leeches are used to prevent blood clotting after severe wounding or plastic surgery, and for varicose veins. The Chinese use dried leeches to mobilize congealed blood after injury or thrombosis, as well as for amenorrhea, and Unani medicine gives them for hemorrhoids and inflammation of the throat and urinary tract.
PREPARATIONS: Powder, sometimes made into a paste with honey or oil.

Homo sapiens ⚥
MAN

Blood, urine, and placentas from the human body all provide medicines that are widely used. Blood's most obvious application in medicine is for blood transfusions, but particular elements such as clotting factors are also extracted. Generally regarded as unclean waste, urine actually contains many useful substances, including hormones, minerals, and vitamins, and millions of people daily take medicine or contraceptives made from substances extracted from human or animal urine. In India, urine therapy is a long established, if minority, practice. The placenta is the channel through which blood, oxygen, nutrients, and waste products travel between a pregnant woman and her fetus. In several societies, the expelled placenta, or afterbirth, has traditionally been eaten by a new mother, as it is by many mammals, because of the goodness it is thought to contain. Saliva is a primitive do-it-yourself medicine that is often applied instinctively to cuts and sores.

PARTS USED: Whole blood or separated fractions; whole urine or extracted substances; fresh saliva; whole placenta or extracted hormones; bone marrow and organs.
ACTIVE INGREDIENTS: *Blood*: immunoglobulins, albumin, gamma globulin, substances that help clotting such as Factor VIII and thrombin. *Urine*: estrogen, gonadotrophic, luteinizing, and follicle-stimulating hormones, mineral salts, and vitamins. *Saliva*: starch-digesting enzymes. *Placenta*: gonadotrophic hormones.

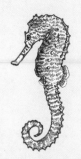

Hippocampus kelloggi

ACTIONS: *Blood products*: prevent hemorrhage, help prevent infection; *urine*: nutrient, hormonal; *placenta*: hormonal; *saliva*: mildly antiseptic.

MEDICINAL USE: Apart from transfusions, the main use of blood preparations is to arrest hemorrhaging, for example, factor VIII in hemophiliacs. Gamma globulin is given to reduce the risk of hepatitis. Extraction of sex and pituitary hormones from human urine started in China in the 2nd century BC. Today, hormones from urine or placenta are given to induce ovulation in women, to treat undescended testes in young men, and for infertility treatment. In Chinese medicine, the clear urine of healthy boys under 12 years is given for tuberculosis and chronic cough, and dried placenta is taken as a general tonic, especially for blood and energy deficiency, for sterility, and for impotence. Bone marrow and organs such as kidneys, livers, and hearts are used in transplant operations.

PREPARATIONS: Liquid blood, urine, pharmaceutical preparations, dried whole placenta, fresh saliva.

Hordeum vulgare (Graminae) 🌿
BARLEY

Barley was one of the first crops ever farmed; records of it go back to neolithic times. As well as being a staple cereal, barley has long been used as a medicine for all manner of internal and external afflictions. It was also used as a nutritive for, in Culpeper's words, "persons troubled with fevers, agues, and heats in the stomach." Native to the East, barley is an annual grass with distinctive ears of grain that have long, stout bristles.

PARTS USED: Polished grains, germinating seeds.

ACTIVE INGREDIENTS: Indole alkaloid, gramine; proteins; B vitamins.

ACTIONS: Nutritive; soothes internal body surfaces.

MEDICINAL USE: Used in convalescence, especially after diarrhea or bowel disease. The Chinese prescribe it for loss of appetite, poor digestion, and fullness in the abdomen.

PREPARATIONS: Grains, decoction, malt extract.

Humulus lupulus (Cannabinaceae) 🌿
HOPS

Hops were first used in beer making in 14th century Flanders. They reached Britain two centuries later, where they were used in medicine for insomnia and for calming nervous stomachs. Native to Europe, North America, and parts of Asia, the hop plant is a perennial climber with heart-shaped, finely toothed, lobed leaves and male and female flowers on separate plants in late summer. The male flowers grow in loose bunches and the female flowers are yellowish green, conelike catkins.

PARTS USED: Female flowers or cones.

ACTIVE INGREDIENTS: Volatile oil containing humulene, myrcrene, and caryophylline; bitter substances, humulone, and lupulones; flavonols, including quercitin and astragalin; resin; tannins; traces of estrogenlike substances.

ACTIONS: Sedative; tranquilizer; promotes sleep; reduces muscle tension and spasms; increases urine production; bitter (digestive stimulant).

MEDICINAL USE: Given to promote restful sleep and for relief of nervous intestinal conditions, including irritable bowel syndrome. Hops are also an anaphrodisiac for men.

PREPARATIONS: Dried, tablets, tincture, extract.

Hydrastis canadensis (Ranunculaceae) 🌿
GOLDENSEAL, ORANGE ROOT

Used by Native Americans as a dye as well as a medicine, goldenseal became so popular with European settlers that it was soon overpicked and now has to be specially cultivated. It was used medicinally for vaginal inflammation and external ulceration or wounds; the efficacy of these uses has been confirmed by recent research. A native of North America, it is a perennial with a large rhizome and a flowering stem with two five-lobed, serrated leaves. Insignificant flowers appear in spring and develop into raspberrylike fruit.

PARTS USED: Rhizome and root.

ACTIVE INGREDIENTS: Alkaloids including hydrastine, berberine, and canadine; volatile oil; resin.

ACTIONS: Astringent to and promotes healing of the gut wall and mucous membranes; digestive stimulant; increases the flow of bile.

MEDICINAL USE: Used as a douche for vaginal infections like thrush and trichomonas. Also given internally for intestinal inflammation, including gastritis and peptic ulcers, as a mouthwash for ulcers and inflamed gums, and externally for wounds and eruptions.

PREPARATIONS: Decoction, tablets, tincture.

CAUTION: **Should be avoided during pregnancy and by people with high blood pressure because it can cause the muscles of the uterus and the blood vessels to contract.**

Hyoscyamus niger (Solanaceae) 🌿☠
HENBANE, DEVIL'S EYE,
STINKING NIGHTSHADE

A centuries-old medicine, henbane was also a famous poison: Shakespeare had Hamlet's father die from henbane juice poured into his ear. Its medicinal uses ranged from a painkiller to a head lice killer and all parts of the plant were used, in the form of a cigarette, dried herb, or juice. Native to Europe but naturalized in the Americas and Australasia, it is an annual or biennial. It has long, sticky leaves and brown or yellow flowers with purple veins in summer.

PARTS USED: Leaves, particularly from the flowering plant.

ACTIVE INGREDIENTS: Tropane alkaloids, particularly hyoscyamine and hyoscine.

ACTIONS: Reduces muscle tension and spasms; sedative; blocks cholinergic nervous system.

MEDICINAL USE: Used to relieve bronchial spasm or asthma, colic, or excessive use of purgatives, and

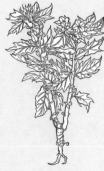

Hyoscyamus niger

to prevent motion sickness. The homeopathic remedy *Hyoscyamus* is prescribed for twitching, coughs, sensitive skin, and excited or obsessional behavioral problems.

PREPARATIONS: Herbal cigarettes, tincture, homeopathic remedies.

CAUTION: Use only under the guidance of a qualified practitioner.

Hypericum perforatum (Hyperaceae)
ST. JOHN'S WORT, GOUTWEED

The Greek word *hypericon*, meaning "due to an apparition," reflects the legendary magical properties of this plant, which included chasing away the devil. The common name comes from the fact that its yellow petals turn red when crushed and that it flowers around June 24th, the date St. John was beheaded. A native of Europe and Asia but widely naturalized, it is a perennial with woody stems, tiny oblong leaves that have transparent oil glands, and clusters of five-petalled, yellow flowers in early summer.

PARTS USED: Dried tops, including flowers.
ACTIVE INGREDIENTS: Essential oil containing caryophyllene, pinene, limonene, and myrcene; hypericins; flavonoids; resin.
ACTIONS: Sedative; astringent; relieves anxiety; antidepressant; anti-inflammatory; antiseptic.
MEDICINAL USE: Used internally to treat excitability and mild anxiety, particularly when associated with depression, and externally for wounds, burns, and infections. Used in homeopathy (*Hypericum*) for nerve injury and bedsores. Used in Chinese medicine for acute hepatitis, appendicitis, snakebites, boils, and abscesses.
PREPARATIONS: Infusion, red oil made from flowers, tincture, cream, homeopathic remedies.

Hyssopus officinalis (Labiatae)
HYSSOP

An ancient insecticide, hyssop was strewn on floors and shelves to repel insects, and has been used to kill head lice and internal worms, as well as for its more traditional role of easing colds and coughs. Native to Europe and western Asia, it prefers alkaline soil in a sunny position. It is a highly aromatic perennial with thin, pointed leaves covered in fine hairs and small, blue flowers in late summer.

PARTS USED: Whole herb.
ACTIVE INGREDIENTS: Volatile oil containing pinene, pinocamphone, camphor, thujone, and linalool; terpenoids, including marrubiin, oleanolic, and ursolic acids; flavonoids; tannins.
ACTIONS: Induces sweating; expectorant; relieves gas and colic; affects the lungs; sedative.
MEDICINAL USE: Given for bronchitis, chronic nasal catarrh, coughs, and colds. In Chinese medicine, giant hyssop is used for wounds, vomiting, diarrhea, and angina.
PREPARATIONS: Infusion, tincture.

Ilex paraguariensis (Aquifoliaceae)
YERBA MATÉ, PARAGUAY TEA, JESUIT'S TEA

Contrary to popular belief, maté is rich in caffeine. It has been used since ancient times by Native South Americans as a stimulating drink, particularly during arduous walks in the Andes. Native to South America, it is a tree growing to 18 feet and has shiny, serrated leaves and small, white flowers that turn into red berries.

PARTS USED: Leaves.
ACTIVE INGREDIENTS: Alkaloids, including caffeine; tannins; volatile oil.
ACTIONS: Central nervous system stimulant; reduces muscle tension and spasms; increases urine production.
MEDICINAL USE: Given for nervous headaches associated with fatigue and to reduce the appetite in people who overeat.
PREPARATIONS: Infusion.

Inula helenium (Compositae)
ELECAMPANE, SCABWORT, HORSEHEAL

Said to be named after Helen of Troy, *I. helenium* was well known to the ancient Greeks and Romans, who used it as a digestive tonic after indulgent feasting. It is native to Europe, where it grows in damp pastures and on roadsides, and used to be grown in European gardens for use as a medicine and confection. A perennial with a deep taproot and hairy stems, it has large, egg-shaped leaves and, in late summer, many slender, bright yellow flower heads.

PARTS USED: Root.
ACTIVE INGREDIENTS: Inulin; volatile oil containing sesquiterpene lactones, especially alantolactones.
ACTIONS: Stimulating expectorant; induces sweating; digestive; stops the growth of bacteria.
MEDICINAL USE: Given for bronchial and other respiratory conditions where resistant catarrh produces a persistent cough, for coughs in tuberculosis, and for irritating coughs in children. Used for similar conditions by Chinese physicians, who also prescribe it for worms.
PREPARATIONS: Infusion, tincture.

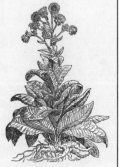

Inula helenium

Iris versicolor (Iridaceae)
BLUE FLAG, WILD IRIS, LIVER LILY

The American pharmacopoeia used to include this plant, a remedy for stomach complaints learned from the Native Americans. It is native to North America, growing in moist, swampy soil, but has been introduced elsewhere for medicinal and ornamental purposes. The thick rhizome supports a stem sheathed in sword-shaped leaves. Bright blue-violet flowers appear in early to midsummer.

PARTS USED: Rhizome.
ACTIVE INGREDIENTS: Volatile oil; iridin; salicylic and isophthalic acids; resin.
ACTIONS: Laxative; increases bile flow and urine production; circulatory and lymphatic stimulant.

MEDICINAL USE: Particularly used for skin eruptions, for which it is given both internally and as a poultice. It is also used for biliousness associated with constipation and disturbances of the liver.

PREPARATIONS: Decoction, tincture, tablets.

Juniperus communis (Coniferae)
JUNIPER

Most familiar as a flavoring in gin, juniper has been used medicinally since the time of ancient Greek and Arab physicians. An oddity of the plant is that the small berries it produces take two years to ripen. Native to southern Europe, which remains the source of most commercial juniper berries, it is an evergreen tree with flat, needlelike leaves, tiny flowers in late summer, and small, green berries that ripen to black.

PARTS USED: Berries.

ACTIVE INGREDIENTS: Volatile oil containing myrcene, sabinene, pinene, limonene, and cineole; condensed tannins; bitter principle; flavonoids.

ACTIONS: Urinary antiseptic; increases urine production; relieves gas and colic; stimulates the muscles of the uterus.

MEDICINAL USE: Used to treat colic, rheumatism, and urinary tract infections, particularly cystitis.

PREPARATIONS: Dried berries, tincture.

CAUTION: **Avoid during pregnancy or if kidney disease is suspected.**

Kaolin ☙
HYDRATED ALUMINUM SILICATE

Named after the Kao-Ling mountain in northern China, where it was first identified, this fine white clay was introduced to Europe in 1712 and was later mined worldwide for use in porcelain. It is also widely known as an antidiarrheal pharmaceutical preparation.

PARTS USED: Cleaned clay.

ACTIVE INGREDIENTS: Aluminum silicate.

ACTIONS: Absorbs toxic substances; anti-inflammatory.

MEDICINAL USE: Widely used as a basis for medicinal dusting powders. Also given internally in orthodox medicine for diarrhea, to absorb harmful substances in the intestines, and increase the bulk of feces, and applied externally as a poultice to reduce swelling and pain.

PREPARATIONS: Suspension, dusting powder, poultice.

Laccifer lacca/Coccus lacca ⚕
SHELLAC, LACCA

Shellac is a reddish resin that the female lac-insect exudes over twigs to build a trap in which to lay and hatch her eggs. East and West have their own species of the lac-insect; many Westerners come into daily contact with shellac as an ingredient of varnishes, cake glazes, hair sprays, wood fillers and polishes, as well as in medicines.

Collected twigs, still carrying the crimson bodies of the lac-insect, are known as stick-lac and provide a crimson dye before the resin is separated off for other purposes.

PARTS USED: Flakes of resin.

ACTIVE INGREDIENTS: Resinoltannols of aleuritic acid; erythrolaccin; lacconic acid.

ACTIONS: Anti-inflammatory; anti-infective; stimulates the stomach.

MEDICINAL USE: Regarded by Chinese physicians as an aid to healing, particularly for bleeding gums, excess menstrual bleeding, and fainting after childbirth. Unani physicians give it for blood, kidney, and liver disorders. In orthodox medicine, it is commonly used to coat tablets.

PREPARATIONS: Separated resin, melted and filtered.

Lachesis mutus ⚕
BUSHMASTER SURUCUCU SNAKE

The rattle of this species of the rattlesnake family is outstandingly loud. At up to 9 feet long, it is one of the most alarming snakes of Central and South America. Apart from the employment of its venom to make an antidote for its bite, this snake is used medicinally by homeopaths, who consider it a remedy ideally suited to patients with left-sided symptoms.

PARTS USED: Venom.

ACTIVE INGREDIENTS: Not known.

ACTIONS: Not known.

MEDICINAL USE: Given as a homeopathic remedy (*Lachesis*) for headaches, epilepsy, palpitations, angina, appendicitis, painful swollen throats, menstrual cramps, and boils and abscesses.

PREPARATIONS: Homeopathic remedies.

Lactobacillus acidophilus & Streptococcus thermophilus ⚕
YOGURT CULTURES

Yogurt is milk that has been colonized by living bacteria, traditionally those listed above. Its modern association with good health follows reports of large scale consumption by Eastern European communities who enjoy unusually long and active lives. Many orthodox doctors still dismiss the possibility of yogurt having any health value beyond the nutritional properties of milk. However, the amount of medical research into the importance of "friendly" bacteria in the digestive system is increasing. Most commercial yogurt companies have replaced the organisms *L. acidophilus* and *S. thermophilus* with ones less likely to survive the human digestive system, and many yogurts are pasteurized after manufacture, a heating process that kills bacteria. It is therefore important that live yogurt is used for medical purposes.

PARTS USED: Live yogurt made with traditional cultures.

ACTIVE INGREDIENTS: Bacteria; B vitamins.

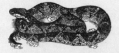

Lachesis mutus

ACTIONS: Antidiarrheal; competes with harmful bacteria in intestines; nutrient.
MEDICINAL USE: The food value of yogurt is often beneficial for those who cannot tolerate ordinary milk. Live bacteria can help restore the microbial balance of the intestines after it has been destroyed by a bout of diarrhea or a course of antibiotic drugs. Yogurt is also applied vaginally for thrush.
PREPARATIONS: Live fresh yogurt, tablets, powder.

Lactuca virosa (Compositae) 🍃
WILD LETTUCE, PRICKLY LETTUCE, LETTUCE OPIUM

Known as poor man's opium, the white latex of this plant was used in the 19th century to adulterate opium. It is, however, much milder than opium and does not disrupt the stomach as much. Wild lettuce has also long been used in cough mixtures as a sedative and cough suppressant. Native to Europe, this biennial plant has a slightly raised rosette of hairy, oval leaves. In the second year of growth, numerous yellow, daisylike flowers appear. The plant has a strong odor and all parts exude a white latex when cut.
PARTS USED: Latex, dried leaves.
ACTIVE INGREDIENTS: The sesquiterpene lactone and lactucin; flavonoids, including quercetin; coumarins.
ACTIONS: Sedative; promotes sleep; mild pain reliever.
MEDICINAL USE: Used to treat bronchitis, irritable coughs, insomnia (particularly in children), anxiety, and restlessness.
PREPARATIONS: Infusion, tincture.
CAUTION: Use only under the guidance of a qualified practitioner, as overdose can produce stupor, coma, and death.

Lavandula angustifolia (Labiatae) 🍃
LAVENDER

Renowned since Roman times as a perfume, and as a flavoring for foods and medicine, lavender is reputed to have many and varied applications. Its current uses, however, are mainly as a flavoring for drugs and as a nervine to treat the nervous system. Native to western Europe near the Mediterranean, it is a woody perennial shrub with narrow, gray-green leaves and blue-violet flowers on spikes in mid- to late summer.
PARTS USED: Flowers.
ACTIVE INGREDIENTS: Volatile oil containing linalyl acetate, linalool, borneol, camphor, and limonene; coumarins; flavonoids.
ACTIONS: Relieves gas and colic; reduces muscle tension and spasms; circulatory stimulant; nerve tonic.
MEDICINAL USE: Given as a general relaxant, especially in baths, and to relieve irritability, exhaustion, and depression. It is also used internally as a digestive tonic and a carminative to relieve flatulence, and externally to relieve tension headaches and arthritic or muscular pain.
PREPARATIONS: Volatile oil, tincture.

Leonurus cardiaca (Labiatae) 🍃
MOTHERWORT, LION'S EAR

The ancient Greeks used motherwort to relieve anxiety in new mothers, whence its common name derives. Research has also shown that the herb is able to calm the palpitations and irregular heartbeats sometimes created by nervous tension and anxiety. A European native, it is perennial with hairy leaves and stems and whorls of pink-blue flowers in midsummer.
PARTS USED: Whole herb.
ACTIVE INGREDIENTS: Iridoid glycosides, including leonuride; diterpenes, including leocardin; flavonoids, including rutin, quercetin, hyperoside, and apigenin.
ACTIONS: Mild stimulant to the uterus; relaxant; reduces muscle tension and spasms; tonic to the heart; mildly lowers blood pressure.
MEDICINAL USE: Used to treat menstrual cramps, particularly when nervous tension is a factor, and to help contract the uterus after birth, so that the placenta is expelled. It is also given for general nervous tension, and for palpitations and tachycardia (an abnormally fast heartbeat). In Chinese medicine, it is prescribed for menstrual problems, raised blood pressure, heart disease, and conjunctivitis.
PREPARATIONS: Infusion, tincture, tablets.

Leptandra virginica/Veronicastrum virginica/Veronica virginica (Scrophulariaceae) 🍃
BLACK ROOT, CULVER'S ROOT, PHYSIC ROOT, BOWMAN'S ROOT

Native to North America and widespread through mountain meadows and open woodlands, blackroot was used by Native Americans as an emetic to cause vomiting in both rituals and medicine. The fresh root is strongly cathartic (empties the bowels) but this property is much reduced in dried roots. A perennial, it grows from a black taproot and has spearlike leaves that grow in whorls resembling a star. Pink, blue, or white flowers appear in late summer on spikelike branches.
PARTS USED: Dried root.
ACTIVE INGREDIENTS: Volatile oil; saponins; bitter principle, lepandrin; tannins.
ACTIONS: Increases the flow of bile; mild laxative.
MEDICINAL USE: Given for constipation associated with signs of liver congestion, jaundice, and cholecystitis (inflammation of the gallbladder).
PREPARATIONS: Tincture.

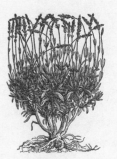
Lavandula angustifolia

Levisticum officinale (Umbelliferae) 🍃
LOVAGE

A popular herb throughout history in both culinary and medicinal arts, lovage is still used as a flavoring in food products and alcoholic beverages. Native to the Mediterranean coast of Europe, it is a perennial with a strong, fleshy root, divided leaves of maple-leaf-like leaflets, and umbrellalike clusters of white flowers in midsummer, followed by flat, brown seeds.

PARTS USED: Root.

ACTIVE INGREDIENTS: Volatile oil containing phthalides; coumarins, including bergapten, coumarin, psoralen, and umbelliferone; beta-sitosterol.

ACTIONS: Aids digestion; reduces muscle tension and spasms; expectorant; antimicrobial.

MEDICINAL USE: Given for flatulent and colicky indigestion, bronchial infections, painful or insufficient menstruation, and as a mouthwash in minor infections. A close relative, *Angelica sinensis*, is used in Chinese medicine for menstrual problems and rheumatic pain.

PREPARATIONS: Tincture.

Linum usitatissimum (Linaceae) 🍃
LINSEED, COMMON FLAX

Linseed was one of the first cultivated plants; records of this date from 5,000 BC. It was used by the Egyptians to make cloth in which to wrap mummies, and the Bible contains many references to the growing and spinning of flax. Now widely cultivated, it is an annual with narrow, green, spearlike leaves and blue, five-petalled flowers in mid- to late summer. Fragile brown capsules containing flattened, shiny seeds follow.

PARTS USED: Seeds.

ACTIVE INGREDIENTS: Fixed oil based mainly on glycerides of linoleic, linolenic, and oleic acids; the glycoside linimarin; mucilage; protein.

ACTIONS: Bulk laxative; soothes internal body surfaces; softens and soothes the skin; inhibits coughing.

MEDICINAL USE: Used internally to treat constipation associated with an abnormally functioning colon, this being one that lacks tone or is spastic, and to relieve dry and irritating coughs. Applied externally as a poultice to draw boils and furunculoses (clusters of boils).

PREPARATIONS: Crushed seed.

Lobelia inflata (Campanulaceae) 🍃
INDIAN TOBACCO, PUKEWEED

Native Americans smoked lobelia to cure asthma and related respiratory problems. The herb was one of the most important to the physiomedical school of herbal medicine that flourished in North America in the 19th century, and it first appeared in Europe in 1829. It is an annual or biennial with hairy, oval to oblong leaves that have a finely toothed margin and blue flowers in the summer, followed by small, round capsules containing two seeds.

PARTS USED: Herb collected during fruiting.

ACTIVE INGREDIENTS: Alkaloids, including lobeline, lobelidine, lobelanine, isolobelanine, and isolobelanidine; chelidonic acid; resin; gum.

ACTIONS: Respiratory stimulant; antiasthmatic; reduces muscle tension and spasms; in large doses causes vomiting.

MEDICINAL USE: Used internally to treat asthma and chronic bronchitis and externally for rheumatic and muscular inflammation. It can help alleviate nicotine withdrawal symptoms and is contained in some over-the-counter antismoking products.

PREPARATIONS: Herbal cigarettes, dried herb, tincture, over-the-counter products.

CAUTION: **Use only under the guidance of a qualified practitioner.**

Lonicera caprifolium (Caprifoliaceae) 🍃
ITALIAN WOODBINE

Dioscorides, in the 1st century AD, recommended honeysuckle for asthma and diseases of the spleen and liver. Culpeper, however, who had to work hard to find uses for the plant, said, "Take a leaf and chew it in your mouth and you will quickly find it likelier to cause a sore throat than cure it." Native to Europe but grown around the world, it is a climbing deciduous shrub with oval leaves and, in midsummer, trumpet-shaped, fragrant flowers, followed by yellow to red berries.

PARTS USED: Flowers, leaves.

ACTIVE INGREDIENTS: Glycosides; salicylic acid; mucilage.

ACTIONS: Expectorant; causes vomiting.

MEDICINAL USE: Rarely used now, but it is a gentle expectorant and laxative. In Chinese medicine, it is prescribed for colds, laryngitis, dysentery, food poisoning, boils, and rheumatism.

PREPARATIONS: Dried herb, infusion.

CAUTION: **The berries are poisonous.**

Lophophora williamsii (Cactaceae) 🍃
MESCAL BUTTONS, PEYOTE, ANHALONIUM, DEVIL'S ROOT

This is known as the "sacred mushroom" of the Aztecs but it is actually a small cactus as opposed to a fungus. Its cult use spread throughout the Americas, and mescal buttons are still taken today by some Mexican tribes for their hallucinogenic properties. The cactus is native to Mexico but can be cultivated elsewhere. The plant is only about 1 inch high, has thin stems, or "buttons," and small, pink flowers.

PARTS USED: Dried tops.

ACTIVE INGREDIENTS: Alkaloids, notably mescaline, but also anhalamine, anhalidine, and lophophorine.

ACTIONS: Hallucinogenic; causes vomiting.

MEDICINAL USE: Has been used for a range of conditions, including nervous disorders, asthma, gout, and rheumatism. However, it is not used in medicine today.

PREPARATIONS: Tincture.

CAUTION: **Possession is illegal.**

Lumbricum terrestris ♉
EARTHWORM

The earthworm benefits man by recycling the soil to make it more productive. It is also used in Chinese medicine.

Lophophora williamsii

PARTS USED: Whole worm.
ACTIVE INGREDIENTS: Not known.
ACTIONS: Helps reduce fever; dilates the airways; prevents convulsions; increases urine production.
MEDICINAL USE: Widely used in Chinese medicine for breathing difficulties, coughs, water retention, and fevers, particularly those related to the lungs, and as an antidote to poisons.
PREPARATIONS: Powder.

Lycosa cubensis/Tarentula cubensis ♥
WOLF SPIDER, TARANTULA SPIDER

Although often called tarantulas, wolf spiders come from a completely different but just as fascinating family. They carry their eggs in a ball behind them and navigate by the stars. The *cubensis* species of wolf spider is used in homeopathy.

PARTS USED: Whole spider.
ACTIVE INGREDIENTS: Not known.
ACTIONS: Counters swelling.
MEDICINAL USE: Given by homeopaths (*Tarentula cubensis*) for swellings and abscesses. The trap-door spider (*Cteniza fodiens*) is used in Chinese medicine for similar purposes, particularly for carbuncles and skin ulcers.
PREPARATIONS: *Wolf spider*: homeopathic tablets. *Trap-door spider*: ashed and mixed with lard.

Lytta vesicatoria ♥☠
SPANISH FLY, BLISTER BEETLE

The deadly potential of the Spanish fly led to a murder conviction for the Marquis de Sade, who had given lytta to women because of its reputation as an aphrodisiac. It is actually a soft-bodied beetle with a green or bluish tint; the lethal dose for humans is only 0.03 grams. *Mylabris phalerata* is the Chinese equivalent of blister beetle and is used for similar purposes as lytta. It has hard yellow-and-black wing cases.

PARTS USED: Wing covers of adults, whole beetle.
ACTIVE INGREDIENTS: Cantharidin, a fatty acid.
ACTIONS: Counterirritant; stimulates blood flow to the skin; causes blistering of the skin.
MEDICINAL USE: Because they contain a powerful irritant, Spanish flies are mainly used externally or in homeopathic form (*Cantharis*). Unani and Chinese physicians apply them to the skin to improve circulation, for instance, for local irritations, and to counter infections. Unani medicine also uses them for kidney stones, amenorrhea, or an enlarged spleen. Homeopathic uses also include urinary tract infections.
PREPARATIONS: Powder, plaster, homeopathic remedies.
CAUTION: **Handle with care, can cause blistering.**

Magnetitum ⬡
MAGNETITE, LODESTONE, FERROSOFERRIC OXIDE

One of the most important ores of iron, magnetite is also magnetic; this intrigued scientists of early China, Greece, and Rome and led to its name. Magnetite is richly distributed around the world as shiny black, perfect, eight-sided crystals.

PARTS USED: Whole mineral.
ACTIVE INGREDIENTS: Ferric oxide; ferrous oxide; magnesium oxide; aluminium oxide.
ACTIONS: Sedative; helps liver function.
MEDICINAL USE: Prescribed by the Chinese for tremors or palpitations, including those caused by fear, and for dizziness, blurred vision, vertigo, and asthma.
PREPARATIONS: Powder.

Manganite ⬡
HYDRATED MANGANESE OXIDE

Manganese is essential to health but, as is the case with some other minerals, it is not known why. In animals, manganese deficiency is linked with poor growth and reproduction, defects in the bone formation and nervous systems of offspring, and anemia. Apart from a study showing that diabetics have much lower levels, human deficiency has not been described. Even so, manganese is accepted as essential and is considered necessary for building proteins that carry genetic information from one generation to the next. There is no official RDA but a safe recommended limit is 5mg/day. Manganese is supplied by tea, nuts, whole grains, and dark, leafy vegetables.

PARTS USED: Manganese salts.
ACTIVE INGREDIENTS: Manganese.
ACTIONS: Nutrient.
MEDICINAL USE: Some therapists give manganese to schizophrenics to counteract their high body copper levels and to diabetics to offset their low body levels. Tiny amounts are sometimes added to solutions for patients on parenteral nutrition (nutrition into a vein).
PREPARATIONS: Tablets.

Marrubium vulgare (Labiatae) ♪
WHITE HOREHOUND

One of the oldest and most reliable cough remedies known, white horehound has been used since the time of the Egyptian pharaohs. It is also reputed to be an antidote to various poisons. Native to Europe, where is it widely found on roadsides and waste places, white horehound is a perennial with hairy, square stems and oval, wrinkled, leathery leaves. It has small, white flowers that appear in summer and give way to an urn-shaped receptacle containing tightly packed seeds.

PARTS USED: Whole herb, collected during flowering.
ACTIVE INGREDIENTS: Diterpene lactone, marrubiin; diterpene alcohols, including marrubiol; volatile oil containing alpha-pinene, sabine, camphene, and p-cymol; alkaloids; tannins.
ACTIONS: Stimulating expectorant; bitter tonic; antiseptic; circulatory stimulant; increases the flow of bile.

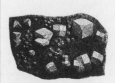

Magnetitum

MEDICINAL USE: Given for catarrhal colds, bronchitis, whooping cough, and poor digestion.
PREPARATIONS: Infusion, tincture.

Matricaria recutita/M. chamomilla (Compositae) ✿
GERMAN CHAMOMILE, WILD CHAMOMILE

Although not the true chamomile (*Chamamaelum nobilis*) in the botanical sense, *M. recutita* closely resembles it in appearance and medical uses. It has been known of since ancient times and has been called the plant's physician because ailing garden plants recover when it is planted close to them. Native to Europe and northern Africa but naturalized in North America, it is a low-growing perennial with finely divided leaves and daisylike flowers.

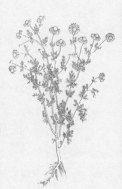

Matricaria recutita/ M. chamomilla

PARTS USED: Flowers.
ACTIVE INGREDIENTS: Volatile oil, containing azulenes, particularly chamazulene, matricine, and alpha-bisabolol oxides A and B; flavonoids, including apigenin, luteolin, and quercetin; coumarins.
ACTIONS: Reduces muscle tension and spasms; sedative; antifungal; antibacterial; relieves pain; promotes wound healing; relieves gas and colic; bitter (digestive stimulant).
MEDICINAL USE: Used internally as a gentle relaxing sedative for adults and children, for gastritis (stomach inflammation) and irritated intestines, for calming a nervous stomach, and to help relieve menstrual cramps, migraines, rheumatism, and gout. It is also applied externally in tea bags to ease allergic dermatitis and eczema, and to help heal burns and weeping wounds. Used in homeopathy (*Chamomilla*) for inner turmoil, anxiety and anger, convulsions, throbbing headache, earache, teething, hacking coughs, menstrual cramps, and diarrhea.
PREPARATIONS: Dried flowers, tincture, infusion, essential oil, cream, homeopathic remedies.

Melaleuca leucadendron (Myrtaceae) ✿
CAJEPUT, SWAMP TEA TREE, PAPERBARK TEA TREE

One of the family of bottlebrush trees, so named because their bright red flowers look like the domestic cleaning tool, cajeput has been used by the Australian Aborigines for 3,000 years. They apply it externally as a local painkiller by rubbing leaves between their hands and then placing them over the affected parts, and also sniff crushed leaves to relieve headaches. Native to Australia and Southeast Asia, it grows in swampy, light soils near the coast. Cajeput is an evergreen tree with slender, hairy leaves, a papery, cream bark, and flowers in summer.

PARTS USED: Twigs, fresh leaves.
ACTIVE INGREDIENTS: Volatile oil containing cineole, terpineol.
ACTIONS: Stimulant; reduces muscle tension and spasms; expectorant; mild pain reliever.
MEDICINAL USE: Given for coughs and colds, to relieve blocked sinuses, catarrh, and asthma, for toothache and headache, and to calm colic and stomach cramps.
PREPARATIONS: Essential oil.

Melissa officinalis (Labiatae) ✿
LEMON BALM, CURE ALL, SWEET BALM

Seen in ancient times as the ultimate remedy for a troubled nervous system, balm was, in one herbal, said to "renew youth, strengthen the brain, relieve languishing nature, and prevent baldness." A native of southern Europe but now a common garden herb throughout the world, it is a perennial with oval, yellowish green leaves which have a strong lemon scent when crushed, and whitish flowers in late summer.

PARTS USED: Whole herb, fresh leaves.
ACTIVE INGREDIENTS: Volatile oil containing citral, linalool, citronellal, nerol, and geraniol; flavonoids; polyphenols, including caffeic and rosmarinic acids.
ACTIONS: Relieves gas and colic; sedative; induces sweating; antiviral.
MEDICINAL USE: Given for anxiety and to relieve nervous tension. It is also useful as a carminative for flatulent digestion. Balm oil and hot water infusions are applied externally for shingles.
PREPARATIONS: Infusion, essential oil, tincture.

Mentha x piperita (Labiatae) ✿
PEPPERMINT

Perhaps the most widely used herbal remedy in the Western world, peppermint is usually taken as a tisane. The Romans and Egyptians used peppermint, but it was not formally recognized as a remedy until the British botanist Ray described a peppery-tasting mint in 1696. A native of Europe but now naturalized in many countries, it is a natural hybrid of watermint and spearmint. This perennial has blackish, square stems and shiny, oval, toothed leaves. Spikes of small, purple flowers appear in summer.

PARTS USED: Whole herb.
ACTIVE INGREDIENTS: Volatile oil containing menthol, menthone, menthyl acetate, pinene, limonene, and cineole; flavonoids, including rutin; rosmarinic acid.
ACTIONS: Reduces muscle tension and spasms; relieves gas and colic; suppresses nausea and vomiting; induces sweating; antiseptic.
MEDICINAL USE: Given to calm digestive problems, indigestion, nausea from overeating and during pregnancy, irritable bowel syndrome, colic, and flatulence. A close relative, *Mentha arvensis*, is prescribed in Chinese medicine for colds, headaches, sore throats, and conjunctivitis.
PREPARATIONS: Infusion, essential oil, tincture.

Menyanthes trifoliata (Menyanthaceae) ✿
BOGBEAN, BUCKBEAN, MARSH TREFOIL

An old remedy for scurvy, rheumatism, and gout, bogbean is now more used as a substitute for *Gentiana lutea* (to which it is related) when a strong bitter is required. The "bean" part of the common name reflects its typical legume-shaped leaves. Native to Europe, where it grows in shallow boggy waters, it is a perennial with a creeping rootstock, cloverlike leaves, and shaggy, white-centered flowers with pinkish edges in midsummer.

PARTS USED: Leaves.
ACTIVE INGREDIENTS: Iridoid glycosides, including foliomenthin and menthiafolin; pyridine alkaloids, including gentianine; coumarins; phenolic acids; vitamin C; tannins; flavonoids.
ACTIONS: Bitter (digestive stimulant); anti-inflammatory; increases urine production.
MEDICINAL USE: Given for rheumatism, indigestion, and anorexia.
PREPARATIONS: Infusion, tincture.

Mirabilitum 🖐

GLAUBER'S SALT, MIRABILITE, SODIUM SULFATE DECAHYDRATE

Mirabilite occurs naturally as colorless or white crystals in deposits from hot springs or salt lakes. It was given the name Glauber's salt in 1668 after Dr. Johann Glauber, a German chemist who described the medicinal properties of the residual sodium sulfate he produced when making hydrochloric acid. He modestly christened it "*sal mirabile*," the wondrous salt.

PARTS USED: Crystals.
ACTIVE INGREDIENTS: Sodium sulfate.
ACTIONS: Purges the bowels.
MEDICINAL USE: In Chinese and orthodox medicine it is prescribed for constipation associated with fever, but only for robust patients and with large amounts of fluid to protect the delicate surface of the intestines. Applied externally by Chinese physicians for red, swollen eyes and ulceration of the mouth, throat, or skin. Given by homeopaths as *Natrum sulphuricum* for water accumulation and swellings.
PREPARATIONS: Powder, pills, decoctions, plasters, injections, homeopathic remedies.

Mitchella repens (Rubiaceae) 🌿

PARTRIDGEBERRY, SQUAW VINE, TWINBERRY

A Native American remedy, partridgeberry was taken by women in the last weeks of pregnancy to make childbirth easier. A native of eastern North America, this small perennial herb has bitter-tasting oval leaves and small, white flowers in summer that give way to red berries.

PARTS USED: Whole herb.
ACTIVE INGREDIENTS: Saponins; mucilage; tannins.
ACTIONS: Aids contraction of the uterus during childbirth; astringent; relaxes the uterus; nerve tonic.
MEDICINAL USE: Given to ease the pain of labor, for menstrual cramps or amenorrhea, and for nervous exhaustion and irritability.
PREPARATIONS: Infusion, tincture.

Montmorillonite 🖐

FULLER'S EARTH

Montmorillonite is a soft rock named after Montmorillon in France, where there are rich deposits. With silica it makes fuller's earth, a name that comes from the use of the clay to "full" cloth, the process of treading cloth with the powdered rock to cleanse and thicken it.

PARTS USED: Rock, ground and cleaned.
ACTIVE INGREDIENTS: Aluminum silicate.
ACTIONS: Absorbent.
MEDICINAL USE: Applied externally in powders when a drying effect is wanted, for example, in weeping skin conditions. Given after poisoning to help absorb harmful substances.
PREPARATIONS: Powder.

Ocimum basilicum (Labiatae) 🌿

SWEET BASIL

Sweet basil is a native of India, where it is revered as a sacred plant. This may be due to its properties as an insect repellent; it keeps disease-carrying flies and mosquitoes away from where it grows. Sweet basil has been cultivated as a culinary herb in Mediterranean countries for centuries. A highly aromatic annual with smooth, slightly curved, green or red leaves, it produces small white flowers in midsummer, followed by small, oval, black seeds.

PARTS USED: Whole herb.
ACTIVE INGREDIENTS: Volatile oil containing linalool, estragole, cineol, borneol, eugenol, and gerianol; phenolic acids; vitamins A and C.
ACTIONS: Aromatic; relieves gas and colic; expels intestinal worms; antibacterial.
MEDICINAL USE: Used mainly for problems of digestion. The oil is also applied externally to treat acne.
PREPARATIONS: Dried herb, essential oil, tincture.

Oenothera biennis (Onagraceae) 🌿

EVENING PRIMROSE, GERMAN RAMPION, FEVER PLANT

The seed oil of evening primrose is particularly rich in a fatty acid called gamma-linolenic acid, which has been shown to be an effective treatment for eczema and premenstrual syndrome, and may also prevent thrombus formation, or blood clotting. A native of North America, it was introduced to Europe via the Padua Botanic Garden in the early 17th century, from where it found its way into gardens all over Europe. Evening primrose is a biennial with a rosette of long, oval leaves in the first year and a vertical hairy stem with spear-shaped, soft leaves in the second year. Yellow flowers, reputed to open only after 6 o'clock in the evening, appear in midsummer.

PARTS USED: Leaves, seed oil.
ACTIVE INGREDIENTS: Fixed oil containing glycerides of linolenic acid and gamma-linolenic acid (GLA).

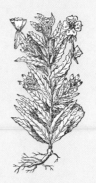

Oenothera biennis

ACTIONS: Prostaglandin precursor.
MEDICINAL USE: The seed oil is used internally to treat eczema, premenstrual syndrome, and heart and vascular disease. The leaves have been used as a poultice on boils and abscesses.
PREPARATIONS: Oil, capsules.

Oleum jacoris aselli ⚕
COD LIVER OIL

Fish liver was recognized as an aid to good health long before it was identified as the richest food source of vitamins A and D, which are needed for the body's defense system and for the absorption of calcium to build healthy bones and teeth. In the north, where less vitamin D is provided by the action of sunlight on the skin, cod and halibut liver oil have been given routinely to guard against deficiency. Recently, other health properties of the oil have been discovered, such as being anti-inflammatory.

PARTS USED: Liver oil.
ACTIVE INGREDIENTS: Vitamins A and D.
ACTIONS: Anti-inflammatory.
MEDICINAL USE: Traditionally, it has been used to treat eczema and arthritis and this has now been validated by medical trials. It is also given as a vitamin supplement.
PREPARATIONS: Liquid, capsules.

Oleum jacoris aselli

Origanum marjorana (Labiatae) ✦
SWEET MARJORAM, ANNUAL MARJORAM, KNOTTED MARJORAM

Closely related to oregano (*O. vulgare*) and other wild marjorams, which have been used as culinary herbs and medicines for centuries, sweet marjoram was used by the ancient Greeks to improve blood flow, and it is still sold at local street markets in Greece as a tea called ditany for digestive problems. Native to northern Africa and central Asia, but now widely distributed, it is a perennial in warmer climates but elsewhere is often grown as an annual. It has square stems, elliptical leaves, and small, pinkish to purple flowers in mid- to late summer.

PARTS USED: Leaves harvested during flowering.
ACTIVE INGREDIENTS: Volatile oil containing sabinine, linalool, terpineol, and eugenol; flavonoids including luteolin and apigenin derivatives; phenolic acids, rosmarinic and caffeic; vitamin A.
ACTIONS: Stimulant; relieves gas and colic; reduces muscle tension and spasms; causes menstruation.
MEDICINAL USE: Used mainly in cooking as a gentle carminative to aid digestion.
PREPARATIONS: Dried herb.

Os draconis ⚕
DRAGON BONES, FOSSILIZED BONES

For the Chinese, dragons represent vitality and good luck, hence their name for these bones (not necessarily dragon bones), which have been fossilized over millions of years.

PARTS USED: Bones.
ACTIVE INGREDIENTS: Calcium carbonate; calcium phosphate.
ACTIONS: Sedative; prevents leakage of fluids.
MEDICINAL USE: A favorite of Chinese medicine for all nervous ailments, liver problems, and discharges ranging from oversweating to abnormal uterine bleeding. The Chinese also apply them externally for persistent sores.
PREPARATIONS: Powder brewed in water.

Ovum ⚕
HEN'S EGG

Every bit of the egg – the yolk, the white, and the shell – has a long history of medicinal use. In addition, the egg's oval shape has given it a mystical role as a treatment for wholeness and harmony.

PARTS USED: Yolk, white, shell, lecithin from yolk.
ACTIVE INGREDIENTS: Mainly in yolk: B complex vitamins, vitamin E, lecithin, vitamin A, choline, inositol, iron, and trace elements.
ACTIONS: *Yolk*: nutritious; *egg white*: astringent; *eggshell*: reduces muscle tension and spasms, discourages discharge.
MEDICINAL USE: Egg yolk, which has a high food value, has long been used by Chinese and Unani physicians as a medicine for the heart. Egg white is given in Chinese medicine to soothe sore throats and by Unani physicians for healing wounds and burns. The shell is taken in Chinese medicine for tuberculosis, inflammation of the stomach lining, and scrofula (tuberculosis of the lymph glands), and in Unani medicine for skin and eye diseases. Lecithin (a waxy fat rich in choline and inositol) is taken by Westerners to break down blood fat deposits and for dementia.
PREPARATIONS: Fresh, powdered shell, lecithin in granules or liquid.

Paeonia officinalis (Ranunculaceae) ✦
PEONY

Named after Paeon, the physician to the Greek gods, peony was used by the ancients in recipes for gallbladder and kidney complaints. At one time, it was said that peony must be picked only at night and then by means of a string attached to a dog, but the herbalist Gerard dismissed these "most superstitious and wicked ceremonies" as trifles. Native to southern Europe but widely distributed, it is a perennial with a large, gnarled rootstock that sends up long stems with compound leaves in spring. The large, attractive flowers have eight crinkled petals that are bright red on opening but fade rapidly to pink.

PARTS USED: Root, petals.
ACTIVE INGREDIENTS: Benzoic acid; alkaloid; essential oil; heteroside.
ACTIONS: Constricts the blood vessels; reduces muscle tension and spasms; stimulates the muscles of the uterus; promotes blood clotting.
MEDICINAL USE: In the past, it was given for convulsions and nervous conditions such as epilepsy. The Chinese use two related peonies

(*P. suffruticosa* and *P. albiflora*) for vascular problems, headaches, and gastric and menstrual pain. Used in homeopathy (*Paeonia*) for itching.
PREPARATIONS: Dried root.

Panax ginseng (Araliaceae) ∮
CHINESE GINSENG, ORIENTAL GINSENG

Ginseng is one of the best known Chinese herbs. Its common name comes from the Chinese *renshen*, meaning man root, after the shape of its thick taproot. The almost magical properties ascribed to ginseng in the West, together with the high price of the best quality herb, have led to much poor quality and diluted ginseng being sold to the public. Korean ginseng is said to be stronger than the Chinese variety. American ginseng, *P. quinquefolium*, lacks some of the key properties of the Oriental species, while *Eleutherococcus senticosus*, or Siberian ginseng, which grows in Russia, has been shown to have similar properties to the Oriental types although it is not a ginseng itself. A perennial with a divided taproot, Oriental ginseng has palm-shaped leaves and small greenish flowers in late summer.

PARTS USED: Root.
ACTIVE INGREDIENTS: Saponin glycosides known as ginsenosides; glycosides; sterols; volatile oil.
ACTIONS: Both stimulant and relaxant on central nervous system; adrenalinlike; improves muscle stamina; heart tonic; lowers blood glucose levels; helps the body adapt to stress.
MEDICINAL USE: Given for debilitated states, particularly after illness or in old age. It is also considered useful for improving concentration and stamina over short periods, and for improving the body's response to stress. The Chinese use ginseng for lack of appetite, forgetfulness, worry, palpitations, insomnia, sweating, and general weakness.
PREPARATIONS: Powdered root, tablets.
CAUTION: **Should not be used for more than 3 weeks by the fit and active and should not be taken when there is acute inflammatory disease, or for depression and anxiety.**

Papaver somniferum (Papaveraceae) ∮
OPIUM POPPY, WHITE POPPY, MAWSEED

Despite all the contemporary publicity about the abuse of the narcotic drug opium, its first recorded use was in medicine. Arabian physicians introduced opium to Europe and India and it was also used by the ancient Greeks and Romans as long ago as the 4th century BC. Two important pharmaceutical drugs, morphine and codeine, are still derived from opium, which is tapped from unripe seed capsules by scratching their surface and harvesting the exuding latex before it has dried. Native to the Middle East and western Asia, the opium poppy is an annual with silvery gray-green leaves and white to lilac flowers in midsummer, followed by globular flat-topped capsules

that contain the poppy seeds. Every part of the plant exudes white latex when scratched, although only that from the capsules is used.

PARTS USED: Latex, leaves.
ACTIVE INGREDIENTS: Alkaloids, especially morphine, codeine, papaverine, and narcotine.
ACTIONS: Narcotic; promotes sleep; relieves pain; reduces muscle tension and spasms; antidiarrheal; inhibits coughing.
MEDICINAL USE: Herbally, it used to be given for diarrhea, to prevent coughs, and to relieve pain, but it is now used as a preoperative relaxant. The extracted morphine is used to relieve severe pain and diarrhea in orthodox medicine, and as the starting material for diamorphine (heroin). Extracted codeine is included in many proprietary cough mixtures and painkillers. The homeopathic remedy (*Opium*) can be given for strokes, alcohol withdrawal symptoms (delirium tremens), irregular breathing, and sneezing.
PREPARATIONS: Tincture, opium extract, pharmaceutical preparations, homeopathic remedies.
CAUTION: **Use only under the guidance of a qualified practitioner. Illegal in the U.S. and Canada.**

Passiflora incarnata (Passifloraceae) ∮
PASSIONFLOWER, MAYPOP, GRANADILLA

The name passionflower is unrelated to romance; it arose because the intricately sculptured corona in the center of the flower resembles Christ's crown of thorns. A native of North America, passionflower is grown throughout the world, thriving on rich soils in sunny positions. It is a perennial vine with a woody stem and three-lobed, serrated leaves. Its flowers are cream with purple centers and give way to orange oval fruit containing seeds in a scented pulp.

PARTS USED: Leaves.
ACTIVE INGREDIENTS: Alkaloids, including passiflorine; flavonoids, including saponarin, vitexin, isovitexin, orientin, and iso-orientin; maltol; sterols.
ACTIONS: Sedative; promotes sleep; reduces musele tension and spasms; lowers blood pressure; relieves pain.
MEDICINAL USE: Used as a nonaddictive remedy for restlessness, insomnia, and irritability. It is also given to relieve muscle spasms in conditions such as asthma and intestinal spasms caused by nervous states, such as irritable bowel syndrome.
PREPARATIONS: Infusion, tablets, tincture.

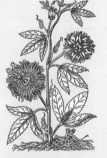

Passiflora incarnata

Perna canaliculata ∯
GREEN-LIPPED MUSSEL

Gaining its name from the handsome green streaks that run along its opening edges, this large mussel is found only off the coast of New Zealand, where it is farmed by "seeding" baby mussels on long ropes that dangle from rafts in deep inlets. The medicinal use of these mussels, which began only 30 years ago, has been controversial but is now more established.

PARTS USED: Gonads.

ACTIVE INGREDIENTS: Not identified but thought to be mucopolysaccharides.

ACTIONS: Anti-inflammatory.

MEDICINAL USE: Taken for both rheumatoid arthritis and osteoarthritis.

PREPARATIONS: Powder in capsules.

Petroselinum crispum

(Umbelliferae)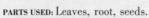

PARSLEY, PERSIL

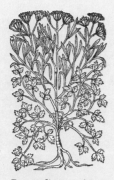

Petroselinum crispum

The Greeks did not eat parsley but revered it as a sacred herb of the gods. Culpeper recommended the herb for stomach, kidney, and menstrual problems, for which it is still used. Native to southern Europe, parsley is a biennial with a deep taproot and divided leaves, which are curled or flat, depending on the variety. Creamy white, umbrellalike clusters of flowers appear in the summer of the second year, followed by small, ribbed, football-shaped fruit.

PARTS USED: Leaves, root, seeds.

ACTIVE INGREDIENTS: Volatile oil containing apiol, myristicin, limonene, eugenol, pinene, and terpinene; coumarins, including bergapten, xanthotoxin, and psoralen; flavonoids, including apiin, lueolin, and glycosides of apigenin and luteolin; vitamins A and C.

ACTIONS: Relieves gas and colic; reduces muscle tension and spasms; promotes bowel movements; increases urine production; stimulates menstruation; antirheumatic; antimicrobial; stimulates milk production.

MEDICINAL USE: Given for urinary tract infections, kidney stones, rheumatic complaints, and poor digestion with intestinal spasms and flatulence. It is also used to help the uterus recover after birth and promote the flow of breast milk.

PREPARATIONS: Infusion, decoction of dried root, fresh leaves, tincture.

CAUTION: **Seeds and leaves should be avoided during pregnancy.**

Phosphorus

Poisonous, yet essential to man, phosphorus is a nonmetallic waxy mineral that is needed for the development of bones and teeth. It also plays a part in converting food into energy and is present in the genetic material that carries inherited characteristics from one generation to the next. The mineral is abundant in so many foods that no shortage is thought likely. However, it is a widely used homeopathic remedy.

PARTS USED: Phosphates.

ACTIVE INGREDIENTS: Phosphorus.

MEDICINAL USE: Homeopaths give the remedy *Phosphorus* for throat and lung disorders, including bronchitis, dry coughs, tonsillitis, hoarseness, laryngitis, and loss of voice. They also use it for tinnitus (ringing in the ears), vomiting, and recurrent sties.

PREPARATIONS: Homeopathic remedies.

Phytolacca decandra/P. americana

(Phytolaccaeae)

POKE ROOT, POKEWEED, AMERICAN NIGHTSHADE

The name poke root is an Americanization of the original Native American name. The herb was used originally to treat venereal disease, but settlers soon learned of its other valuable effects and it has become a useful herb in herbal medicine. Poke root was introduced to Europe in the 19th century and is now cultivated both there and in North America. A perennial, it has strong smelling, oblong to spear-shaped leaves and white to pink flowers, which are followed by round, soft, purple berries.

PARTS USED: Dried root, berries.

ACTIVE INGREDIENTS: Triterpenoid saponins, the phytolaccosides A, B, C, D, and E; lectins; glycoprotein known as pokeweed mitogen.

ACTIONS: Anti-inflammatory; stimulates the immune system; lymphatic; antirheumatic; kills parasites; antifungal.

MEDICINAL USE: Used to treat rheumatoid arthritis and similar autoimmune diseases, inflammatory diseases of the respiratory system, conditions where the lymphatic system needs stimulating, and skin diseases. Given homeopathically (*Phytolacca*) for shooting pains, dizziness on standing, pain in the eyes, sore throats, earache, stiff neck, hip pain, nausea, and painful, lumpy breasts. The Chinese prescribe a close relative, *P. acinosa*, for edema (swelling with water retention) and abdominal distension.

PREPARATIONS: Tincture, tablets.

CAUTION: **Large doses may be cathartic and emetic. Use only under the guidance of a qualified practitioner.**

Picrasma excelsa & Quassia amara

(Simaroubaceae)

JAMAICA QUASSIA; BITTER WOOD

Both plants are members of the Quassia family, the name deriving from the Guyanan slave Quassi, who taught Europeans how to use the plant to treat tropical fevers. It is also a useful insecticide against flies and various mites. *P. excelsa* is native to the West Indies and *Q. amara* is native to South America. Tall trees growing to 65 feet, they have spearlike leaves and small greenish flowers in late summer, followed by bunches of small black fruit.

PARTS USED: Wood.

ACTIVE INGREDIENTS: Bitter quassinoids, including quassin and isoquassin (picrasmin); alkaloids.

ACTIONS: Tonic; bitter (digestive stimulant); kills and helps expel worms; antimalarial.

MEDICINAL USE: Used as a general tonic for debilitation, particularly if associated with poor digestion and loss of appetite. It is also given for infestations of amoebae, threadworms, and nematodes (family of worms).

PREPARATIONS: Decoction, tincture.

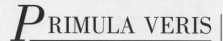
Piscidia piscipula (Leguminosae) 🌿
JAMAICAN DOGWOOD

Jamaican dogwood is poisonous to fish, which has led to a curious fishing technique in South America that involves scattering its crushed leaves and branches in rivers to stun fish so that they can be collected by hand. It also contains rotenone, which is used as an insecticide. Native to Central America, it is a small tree or shrub with longitudinal wings on its pods.

PARTS USED: Bark.
ACTIVE INGREDIENTS: Isoflavones, including lisetin and jamacin; rotenoids, including rotenone, milletone, and isomilletone; piscidic acid; tannins.
ACTIONS: Relieves pain; sedative; reduces muscle tension and spasms.
MEDICINAL USE: Used to treat neuralgia (nerve pain), headache, menstrual cramps, and insomnia.
PREPARATIONS: Tincture.
CAUTION: Use only when prescribed by a qualified practitioner.

Plantago major & P. ovata
(Plantaginaceae) 🌿
PLANTAIN; ISPAGHULA

An ancient folk remedy for healing wounds, relieving coughs, and treating diarrhea, *P. major* used to be associated with superstitions like "three roots will cure one grief, foure another disease, six hanged about the neck are good for another malady," but the herbalist Gerard dismissed these as "ridiculous toyes." In India, the seeds of the related species, *P. ovata*, are used as an effective bulk laxative known as isbogool, while in orthodox medicine the seed husks, known as ispaghula, are used for the same purposes. Native to Europe, plantain thrives on rich wastelands and has travelled the world as a weed. It is a perennial with slightly hairy leaves and a spike of small greenish flowers with tiny purple anthers from midsummer.

PARTS USED: Leaves, seeds.
ACTIVE INGREDIENTS: *P. major*: iridoids, including acubin; flavonoids, including apigenin, luteolin, scutellarin, and baicalein; tannins; organic acids, fumaric and benzoic. *P. ovata*: mucilage.
ACTIONS: *P. major*: soothes internal body surfaces; astringent; expectorant; increases urine production. *P. ovata*: laxative; antidiarrheal.
MEDICINAL USE: Plantain is used in urinary tract infections such as cystitis, in catarrhal conditions of the respiratory tract, and locally for hemorrhoids. It is prescribed in Chinese medicine for a range of conditions, including urinary tract infections, kidney stones, conjunctivitis, and inflammation of the prostate gland. Ispaghula is used in herbalism and Ayurvedic and orthodox medicine for chronic constipation and diarrhea.
PREPARATIONS: *P. major*: infusion, cream, tincture. *P. ovata*: dried seeds or their husks, powder.

Plexaura species 🦑
SEA WHIP CORAL

The sway of these branching, treelike yet stony corals has earned them the zoological name of *Gorgonia*, after the Gorgon Medusa of Greek mythology, whose "hair," made of writhing snakes, turned onlookers to stone. Sea whip coral can grow up to six feet tall in the coral reefs of warm seas throughout the world. Researchers in the West have been investigating it as a source of prostaglandins, chemicals that occur naturally in the body and control many of its functions.

PARTS USED: Outer layers.
ACTIVE INGREDIENTS: Prostaglandins; calcium carbonate.
ACTIONS: Astringent; stops bleeding from external wounds; detoxicant; tonic.
MEDICINAL USE: In orthodox medicine, prostaglandins are given to stimulate many body functions, such as contraction of the uterus during labor. Unani medicine values red coral (*Corallium rubricum*) for a wide range of illnesses, including epilepsy, palpitations, gastric disorders, kidney stones, sexual problems, and general debility. Externally, Unani physicians apply coral ash as a tooth powder, for earache, and as a surma (paste) for eye disorders.
PREPARATIONS: Extracted prostaglandins, powder, ash, paste.

Potentilla erecta/P. tormentilla
(Rosaceae) 🌿
TORMENTIL, BLOODROOT, EWE DAISY

The name tormentil comes from the Latin *tormina*, meaning colic, which was what the herb was traditionally used for in the 16th century. The whole plant is highly astringent and was also used as a therapeutic tooth powder to ease bleeding and infected gums. Native to northern Europe and west Asia, it thrives in lowland areas on damp acid soils. It is a perennial with a thick red-centered rootstock, five-lobed serrated leaves, and bright yellow flowers in summer.

PARTS USED: Root, whole herb.
ACTIVE INGREDIENTS: Tannins; red pigment, phlobaphene.
ACTIONS: Astringent.
MEDICINAL USE: Used internally to treat gastritis (stomach inflammation) and diarrhea, as a mouthwash for gingivitis (inflamed gums) and throat infections, and as a vaginal douche in leukorrhea (excessive white vaginal discharge).
PREPARATIONS: Decoction of root, infusion, tincture.

Primula veris/P. officinalis
(Primulaceae) 🌿
COWSLIP, PAIGLE, ARTHRITICA

According to folklore, cowslips first grew from the ground where St. Peter dropped his keys, and this is recorded in the French, German, and old English names (*clef de Saint Pierre, Schlüsselblumen,* and key of

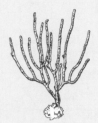

Plexaura species

heaven respectively). The name cowslip, on the other hand, derives from the old English name, cowslop, because the plant used to grow best in meadows frequented by herds of cows. It was given in the Middle Ages to relieve headaches and insomnia. Native to northern Europe, it can be found on alkaline soils but it is becoming rare. Cowslips are perennial with a rosette of oval, wrinkled leaves and large yellow flowers that appear in early spring.

PARTS USED: Dried petals.
ACTIVE INGREDIENTS: Saponin glycosides based on triterpene aglycones, including primulic acid, primulaveroside, and primveroside; volatile oil; tannins; flavonoids, including luteolin, apigenin, kaempferol, and quercetin; phenolic glycosides.
ACTIONS: Stimulating expectorant; sedative; reduces muscle tension and spasms.
MEDICINAL USE: Given to relieve excitability and insomnia, bronchitis, and whooping cough.
PREPARATIONS: Infusion, tincture.

Prunella vulgaris (Labiatae)
SELF HEAL, HEAL ALL

In the Middle Ages, self heal was considered one of the best wound healing remedies. And the herbalist Gerard said that, together with its relative bugle (*Ajuga reptans*), "In all the world there are not two better wound herbs, as has often been proved." Native to Europe, it is now naturalized in many regions. Self heal is a perennial with a creeping rhizome, square stems, and oblong leaves that have sharply toothed margins and a shiny dark green surface. Its flowers are violet, grow in tight spikes, and appear from midsummer.

PARTS USED: Whole herb.
ACTIVE INGREDIENTS: Triterpenes derived from ursolic, betulinic, and oleanolic acid; tannins.
ACTIONS: Astringent; promotes wound healing.
MEDICINAL USE: Used as a styptic to stop bleeding from external wounds and also given internally for bleeding, ulcers, and sore throats. Chinese medicine prescribes it for high blood pressure, conjunctivitis, edema (swelling with water retention), abscesses, and swellings.
PREPARATIONS: Fresh herb, infusion, poultice, tincture.

Prunus domestica (Rosaceae)
PRUNE, PLUM

This fruit dates back to Roman times. Today, the medicinal properties of prunes are taken for granted and the fruit is often included in the Western diet to relieve constipation. Native to Europe and Asia, *P. domestica* is a deciduous tree with smooth, peeling bark and oval leaves. Clusters of pink to white flowers appear in the spring, followed by fleshy, stone-containing fruit, which ripen with a deep purple skin and yellow to brown flesh.

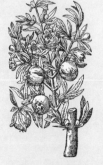

Punica granatum/ P. domestica

PARTS USED: Fruit.
ACTIVE INGREDIENTS: Sugars; malic acid; pectin.
ACTIONS: Laxative; soothes internal body surfaces.
MEDICINAL USE: An ideal nutritive laxative for people with frail and nervous bowel function.
PREPARATIONS: Dried fruit.

Prunus serotina (Rosaceae)
WILD CHERRY, BLACK CHERRY

Wild cherry bark has been included in cough syrups for centuries. Several other *Prunus* species have been used in medicines, but wild cherry is still one of the most useful in contemporary herbal medicine. Widely distributed throughout North America, it is a large tree with oval leaves and clusters of white flowers in spring. The bark is smooth, red-brown, and shiny, and has a bitter, astringent taste.

PARTS USED: Bark.
ACTIVE INGREDIENTS: Cyanogenetic glycoside, prunasin; coumarins; tannins; resin.
ACTIONS: Inhibits coughing; sedative; astringent.
MEDICINAL USE: Used in cough syrups for irritable and unproductive coughs and has been given for digestive problems. Chinese physicians prescribe *P. yedoensis* for coughs.
PREPARATIONS: Syrup, tincture.

Pteria margaritiferia
PEARL

Pearls form as a result of an oyster's, clam's, or mussel's efforts to protect itself from foreign bodies, often parasites, that get inside the shell. The animal completely encloses the enemy in several layers of the same pearly substance that lines the shell. The pearls used medicinally are from sea- rather than freshwater shells.

PARTS USED: Whole pearl.
ACTIVE INGREDIENTS: Calcium carbonate; magnesium carbonate; silica.
ACTIONS: Sedative; helps liver function.
MEDICINAL USE: Chinese physicians prescribe pearl for spasms, convulsions, headache, and insomnia.
PREPARATIONS: Powder.

Punica granatum/P. domestica (Punicaeae)
POMEGRANATE

A fruit mentioned frequently in the Bible and said to have originated in the Garden of Eden, pomegranate was featured in the decoration of King Solomon's temple. It is a common fruit in the eastern Mediterranean and Middle East, where it is taken as an aperitif, eaten as a dessert, or made into wine. Native to western Asia but naturalized throughout Asia, the Americas, and East Africa, it is a perennial tree with oval leaves and striking red, waxy flowers in summer. The fruit has a light brown woody skin and contains crimson juice in individual sacs, each containing a large seed.

OSMARINUS OFFICINALIS

PARTS USED: Rind of fruit, bark.
ACTIVE INGREDIENTS: Alkaloids, including pelletierine and isopelletierine; ellagitannins.
ACTIONS: Kills and helps expel worms; astringent.
MEDICINAL USE: Used to expel intestinal worms and to kill amoebae. The bark is used against tapeworms and is also useful as a vaginal douche in leukorrhea (excessive white vaginal discharge).
PREPARATIONS: Dried rind, tincture.

Quartz
SILICON DIOXIDE, SILICA

Quartz is the most common mineral, making up 12 percent of the earth's crust. It takes many forms, from the colorless crystals of common quartz and stonelike flint to the beautiful amethyst, rose quartz, onyx, tiger's eye, and jasper. Common quartz is the main source of silicon dioxide, which is extensively used for such things as optics, electronic silicon chips, glassmaking, and precision instruments. Synthetic rock crystals have been developed for some of these uses.

PARTS USED: Silicon dioxide.
ACTIVE INGREDIENTS: Silicon dioxide.
ACTIONS: Stops bleeding from external wounds.
MEDICINAL USE: Homeopaths give *Silicea* made from flint for debility due to overexertion, and for boils, carbuncles, abscesses, felons, acne, hay fever, sinus problems, and migraine. Silicon dioxide powder is used as a nonactive ingredient in tablets and capsules to give them bulk.
PREPARATIONS: Homeopathic remedies.

Quercus robur (Fagaceae)
ENGLISH OAK

The oak's reputation is as solid as its wood; it has ancient magical properties, has been used for both animal and human nutrition, is used as a dye and in leather tanning, and is one of the best astringent medicines. Many species of oak with similar uses are found around the world. *Q. robur* is native to Europe, North Africa, and west Asia but is associated traditionally with England. The tree can grow to an enormous girth and spread, and a height of up to 130 feet. The bark is smooth in young trees but soon becomes rough and deeply furrowed. The leaves are oval with large lobes, and are often deformed by galls (swellings) caused by insects. Flowers appear in summer, followed by acorns.

PARTS USED: Bark, galls.
ACTIVE INGREDIENTS: Tannins, including phlobatannin, ellagitannins, and gallic acid.
ACTIONS: Astringent.
MEDICINAL USE: Given internally to treat acute diarrhea, applied locally on burns, bleeding or weeping wounds, and hemorrhoids. It is also used as a mouthwash in gingivitis (inflamed gums) and ulcers, and used as a vaginal douche.
PREPARATIONS: Powdered bark, tincture.

Ricinus communis (Euphorbiaceae)
CASTOR BEAN, PALMA CHRISTI

From the 18th century, *Ricinus* was used as a purgative to clear the bowels and, in the early part of the 20th century, it was a common household remedy for upset stomachs and constipation. The Latin name refers to dog ticks and arose because of the shape and markings of the seeds. Native to India but distributed around the world, it is a perennial shrub or tree with palm-shaped leaves. Flowers without petals appear in summer followed by poisonous seeds that are dark brown with light striped markings.

PARTS USED: Seeds, leaves, root.
ACTIVE INGREDIENTS: Fixed oil containing glycerides ricinoleic, isoricinoleic, stearic, and linoleic acids.
ACTIONS: Laxative; purges the bowels.
MEDICINAL USE: Used internally to treat chronic constipation and acute diarrhea, or as an enema to remove compacted feces in constipation. Also included in proprietary skin and eye lotions as an emollient to soften and soothe the skin. In Chinese medicine, the seeds, leaves, and root of castor bean are used for a range of conditions, including gunshot wounds, joint pains, facial paralysis, and constipation.
PREPARATIONS: Oil.
CAUTION: The seeds are extremely poisonous.

Rosa canina (Rosaceae)
DOG ROSE, BRIER ROSE

The perfume and beauty of roses attracted civilizations as far back as the ancient Egyptians and Romans. Rose petals of several species were once used as an astringent but are now mainly used in cosmetics and as flavorings. Today, only the hips of the dog rose are used in medicine. A native of Europe, West Africa, and Asia, the dog rose can be found growing wild on roadsides and waste ground. It is a thorny climber with oval, serrated leaves and strong-smelling, white or pink flowers in summer. The flowers give way to red hips, which are the swollen bases of the flower and not a true fruit.

PARTS USED: Hips.
ACTIVE INGREDIENTS: Ascorbic acid; flavonoids; fruit acids; mucilage.
ACTIONS: Astringent; nutritive.
MEDICINAL USE: Given as a source of vitamin C in debility, colds, and mild infections. It is also used as an astringent for mild diarrhea and gastritis (stomach inflammation). Chinese medicine uses a close relative of dog rose (*R. laevigata*) for chronic dysentery, urinary tract infections, menstrual irregularites, and trauma.
PREPARATIONS: Syrup, infusion.

Rosmarinus officinalis (Labiatae)
ROSEMARY

Grown in gardens since ancient times, rosemary was considered to have mythical powers of protection against evil spirits and

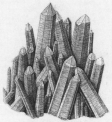
Quartz

121

was used in weddings and funerals. It is still said that rosemary grows strongly in the kitchen gardens of households where the woman rules supreme. A native of the northern shores of the Mediterranean but grown around the world, it is a shrub with leathery, needlelike leaves that have a bluish green hue, and pink to blue flowers from spring to midsummer.

PARTS USED: Leaves.
ACTIVE INGREDIENTS: Volatile oil containing borneol, linalool, pinene, camphéne, cineol, and camphor; flavonoids apigenin, diosmetin, and diosmin; rosmarinic acid; tannins; resin.
ACTIONS: Circulatory stimulant; dilates the blood vessels; anti-inflammatory; astringent; restores the nerves; antiseptic.
MEDICINAL USE: Given for depression, debility, migraines, and skin disease. It is also used when poor liver function is combined with poor circulation, and as a hair rinse for dandruff.
PREPARATIONS: Infusion, juice, tincture.

Rubus idaeus (Rosaceae)
RASPBERRY

Cultivated in Europe since medieval times, raspberry has grown wild there for even longer. The selection and breeding of the raspberry has been prolific and there are now hundreds of varieties, but these differ little from the wild parents. Native to Europe, it is a thorny perennial, with suckers appearing one summer and flowers and fruit the next. The leaves are leathery on top and gray underneath, and the flowers are small, appear in midsummer, and are followed by red cone-shaped fruit.

PARTS USED: Leaves, root.
ACTIVE INGREDIENTS: Flavonoids, including kempferol and quercetin; polypeptides; tannins.
ACTIONS: Astringent; tonic to the pregnant uterus.
MEDICINAL USE: Taken in the last trimester of pregnancy to relax the uterus muscles and facilitate birth. It is also used as a gargle for minor mouth infections and as an eyewash for conjunctivitis. In Chinese medicine, raspberry roots and leaves are prescribed for trauma, bone and muscle pain, amenorrhea, and diarrhea.
PREPARATIONS: Infusion, tincture, tablets.

Rumex crispus (Polygonaceae)
YELLOW DOCK, CURLED DOCK, SOUR DOCK, GARDEN PATIENCE

At the same time in both North America and Europe, related docks were being used as skin cleansing herbs. The ancient Romans also used docks for skin complaints, and the herbalist Gerard said it "purifieth the blood and makes young wenches look fair and cherry like." Native to Europe, yellow dock is now so widespread it is a common weed in many countries. A strong taproot sends up leaves with long stalks and ribbonlike leaves, and whorls of small flowers are produced in midsummer.

PARTS USED: Leaves, root.
ACTIVE INGREDIENTS: Anthraquinone glycosides based on chrysophanol, physcion, and emodin; rumicin; oxalates; tannins.
ACTIONS: Laxative; stimulates nutrition and elimination; increases the flow of bile; tonic.
MEDICINAL USE: Used as a gentle laxative, particularly for chronic constipation. It is also given for chronic skin disease when sluggish liver or bowel function is involved. Given in Chinese medicine for constipation, abdominal cramps, boils, and fungal infections.
PREPARATIONS: Tincture.

Saiga tatarica
ANTELOPE

Many folk traditions have stories of deer and antelopes with miraculous healing powers; these may be connected to millennia of medicinal uses throughout the world. Various species of the two families, *Bovidae* (antelope) and *Cervidae* (deer), are used for a range of quite different ailments. For example, in Chinese medicine antelope horn is used for "hot" conditions and deer horn for "cold" conditions.

PARTS USED: Horn, velvet which grows on horns in spring.
ACTIVE INGREDIENTS: Pantocrin, a hormone in velvet.
ACTIONS: Reduces muscle tension and spasms; helps reduce fever; sedative.
MEDICINAL USE: Chinese physicians prescribe antelope horn for fevers, dizziness, blurred vision, headaches, and convulsions. Russian medicine gives deer velvet as a tonic and to accelerate the healing of wounds and ulcers.
PREPARATIONS: Powder, pills.

Salix alba (Salicaceae)
WHITE WILLOW

An ancient remedy, salix bark was one of the original sources of salicin, the chemical that led to the introduction of aspirin, the most widely used pharmaceutical painkiller. Native to Europe, this graceful tree has a silvery bark and long, pointed, downy leaves. The flowers appear in early summer.

PARTS USED: Bark.
ACTIVE INGREDIENTS: Phenolic glycosides, including salicin, picein, and triandrin with esters of salicylic acid; tannins; coumarins; flavonoids.
ACTIONS: Relieves pain; anti-inflammatory; reduces or prevents fever; tonic.
MEDICINAL USE: Used in the treatment of rheumatic diseases and gout, and in the management of fevers and aches and pains of all kinds. It is also given for food poisoning and dysentery.
PREPARATIONS: Infusion, tincture.

Salvia officinalis (Labiatae)
RED SAGE, GARDEN SAGE, SPANISH SAGE

Sage has been seen as a cure-all throughout history; its generic name comes from the Latin for "to be saved," and it was believed

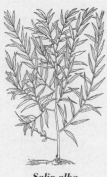

Salix alba

that having sage in the garden meant no illness could prevail. Native to southwest Europe and the northern Mediterranean coast and hinterland, it is a perennial shrub with wrinkled, oval, glandular leaves that can be reddish or green. Violet flowers are produced from late summer to autumn.

PARTS USED: Leaves.
ACTIVE INGREDIENTS: Volatile oil containing thujone, cineole, borneol, and camphor; diterpene bitters; flavonoids, including salvigenin, genkwanin, and luteolin; phenolic acids, including rosmarinic and caffeic acids; estrogenic substances; tannins.
ACTIONS: Astringent; antiseptic; promotes wound healing; reduces salivation and lactation; stimulates the uterus; increases the flow of bile.
MEDICINAL USE: Used as a mouthwash for mouth and throat infections. It is also given to stimulate circulation and digestion in debility, to reduce excessive sweating in anxiety, and to help reduce menopausal symptoms. In Chinese medicine, sage is prescribed for menstrual problems, abdominal pain, insomnia, hepatitis, and hives.
PREPARATIONS: Infusion, tincture.
CAUTION: **Avoid during pregnancy.**

Sambucus nigra (Caprifoliaceae)
BLACK ELDER, EUROPEAN ELDER, PIPE TREE

Elder is a symbol of sorrow and death because of historical reference to its being the wood from which the crucifixion cross was made and the type of tree from which Judas hanged himself. Elder is also associated with magic throughout Europe; it is thought that burning the wood brings all manner of bad luck, but that sprigs hung in houses ward off evil witches. So numerous are its folk medicinal uses that it is called the peoples' medicine chest. A native of Europe and North Africa, where it is common in hedgerows and woods, it is a perennial shrub or small tree with leaves of broad, serrated leaflets and clusters of small cream flowers that have a strong and sweet perfume. Spring flowering is followed by the production of clusters of succulent, deep purple to black berries.

PARTS USED: Flowers, leaves, berries, bark.
ACTIVE INGREDIENTS: Triterpenes, including ursolic acid; fixed oil; flavonoids, including rutin and quercitin; tannins.
ACTIONS: Circulatory stimulant; astringent; induces sweating; expectorant; prevents catarrh; anti-inflammatory; increases urine production.
MEDICINAL USE: The flowers and berries are given to control fever, dry up a runny nose, and remove catarrh from the lungs in colds and flu. The leaves and bark are used as a mouthwash and are applied externally to heal minor burns. In Chinese medicine, elder is prescribed for bone pain, swelling of the legs, muscular spasms, and traumatic injuries.
PREPARATIONS: Infusion, decoction, tincture, mouthwash.

Sanguinaria canadensis
(Papaveraceae)
BLOODROOT, RED ROOT, INDIAN PAINT

Both the Latin and common names of this herb refer to the strong red dye in its root, which was used by Native Americans as a face and cloth dye. Medicinally, it has been used traditionally as an emetic and purgative in the treatment of stomach complaints. A native of North America, where it grows in shaded woods on rich moist soil, it is a perennial with a thick rhizome. Flowers with waxy white petals appear in spring before the leaves, which are as big as a hand and have fingerlike lobes.

PARTS USED: Root.
ACTIVE INGREDIENTS: Alkaloids, including sanguinarine, chelerythrine, berberine, and protopine; red pigment.
ACTIONS: Expectorant; reduces muscle tension and spasms; causes nausea and vomiting; evacuates the bowels; antiseptic.
MEDICINAL USE: Used internally for respiratory and throat infections, applied externally to remove benign skin tumors, and given as snuff for nasal polyps. Extracted sanguinarine is employed as an antiplaque agent in toothpaste and mouthwashes. The homeopathic remedy (*Sanguinaria*) is considered excellent for migraines.
PREPARATIONS: Infusion, tincture, snuff, homeopathic remedies.
CAUTION: **Poisonous, use only under the guidance of a qualified practitioner.**

Scolopendra subspinipes mutilans
CENTIPEDE

Found throughout the world, centipedes have a moderately poisonous bite. This species is an ingredient in several Chinese prescriptions.

PARTS USED: Whole centipede.
ACTIVE INGREDIENTS: D-hydroxylysine.
ACTIONS: Antifungal; sedative; antitumor.
MEDICINAL USE: In Chinese medicine, it is given internally to counter poisoning, and for spasms, convulsions, and lockjaw. It is applied externally to soften and disperse sores and lumps, including cancers, particularly on the neck.
PREPARATIONS: Powder, pills, infusion.
CAUTION: **Avoid during pregnancy.**

Scrophularia nodosa
(Scrophulariaceae)
FIGWORT, THROATWORT, CARPENTER'S SQUARE, SCROFULA PLANT

Used by the Romans for hemorrhoids, figwort also has a longstanding reputation as a treatment for tuberculosis of the lymph glands, and has been used for skin diseases such as psoriasis scd eczema. A European native that thrives in moist loamy soils, figwort is a perennial with square stems, a knotted rootstock, and oval, serrated leaves. It has globular, green or purple flowers in midsummer, followed by egg-shaped fruit.

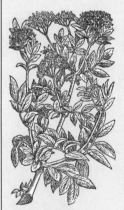

Sambucus nigra

PARTS USED: Whole herb.

ACTIVE INGREDIENTS: Iridoids, including acubin; flavonoids, including diosmin and hesperidin; phenolic acids.

ACTIONS: Increases urine production; stimulates nutrition and elimination; anti-inflammatory; mild pain reliever.

MEDICINAL USE: Given as a gentle circulatory stimulant in people with poor circulation, and for chronic inflammation of the skin, including weeping infections, eczema, and psoriasis. However, it should be avoided by people with heart disease, particularly ventricular tachycardia (an abnormally fast heartbeat). Chinese physicians prescribe figwort species for a wide range of conditions, such as sore throats, constipation, and painful urination.

PREPARATIONS: Infusion, poultice, tincture.

Scutellaria lateriflora, S. baicalensis, & S. galericulata (Labiatae)

SKULLCAP, MAD-DOG WEED, HELMET FLOWER

Skullcap has long had a reputation in North America as a cure for rabies, and in Europe for treating epilepsy. The name skullcap comes from the appearance of its dried calyx, which looks remarkably like a bonnet. A perennial found near water, it has square stems, spearlike serrated leaves, and bright blue-lipped flowers in midsummer.

PARTS USED: Whole herb.

ACTIVE INGREDIENTS: Flavonoid glycoside, scutellarin and scutellarein; flavonoids, including baicalin, baicalein, and wogonin; iridoids; volatile oil; tannins.

ACTIONS: Sedative; restores the nerves; reduces muscle tension and spasms; prevents convulsions.

MEDICINAL USE: Used for anxiety and nervous tension, as a nervous system restorative in long-term depression or nervous exhaustion, and to help reduce the severity and frequency of seizures in epilepsy. Homeopaths have reported success using *Scutellaria* for chronic fatigue syndrome. *S. baicalensis* is used in Chinese medicine for several conditions, including hepatitis, coughs, conjunctivitis, and gonorrhea.

PREPARATIONS: Infusion, tincture, homeopathic remedies.

Selenium

Selenium is an essential trace element that is present in everyday foodstuffs. It is thought to work with vitamin E as an antioxidant, protecting against the destructive effects that oxygen exposure has on cells, and is also a critical nutrient for the nervous system. As selenium is unevenly distributed in different soils, crops vary widely in how much they contain, so it is best to eat varied foods from different sources to ensure a good supply. If eaten in excess, inorganic selenium is harmful, so a safe form is prepared for food supplements by growing yeast on selenium.

PARTS USED: Selenium as selenium sulfide or selenium dioxide.

ACTIVE INGREDIENTS: Selenium; selenium sulfide.

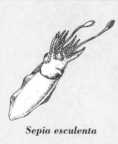

Sepia esculenta

ACTIONS: Nutrient; antioxidant; may make vitamin E more effective; controls dandruff.

MEDICINAL USE: In orthodox medicine, selenium sulfide is applied externally for scalp problems such as dandruff. Internally, selenium is taken by individuals who want to improve their intake of protective antioxidants.

PREPARATIONS: Over-the-counter shampoos, lotions, tablets, and capsules.

Senecio aureus (Compositae)

LIFE ROOT, GOLDEN GROUNDSEL, SQUAW WEED, GOLDEN RAGWORT

Life root was used by Native Americans to treat vaginal discharges but it has recently been found to have wider uses. A native of Canada and the central United States, it thrives in moist soil near water. It is a perennial with heart-shaped leaves at ground level, deeply serrated, spear-shaped upper leaves, and small, yellow, daisylike flowers in early to midsummer.

PARTS USED: Whole herb.

ACTIVE INGREDIENTS: Pyrrolizidine alkaloids, including florosenine, otosenine, floridanine, and senescine; sesquiterpenes.

ACTIONS: Increases urine production; stimulates the pregnant uterus; expectorant; uterus relaxant.

MEDICINAL USE: Given to ease menopausal symptoms such as hot flashes, and nervous and emotional upset. It is also used for amenorrhea and leukorrhea (excessive white vaginal discharge).

PREPARATIONS: Infusion, douche, tincture.

CAUTION: **Large doses may harm the liver. Use only under the guidance of a qualified practitioner. Avoid during pregnancy.**

Sepia esculenta

CUTTLEFISH

Found worldwide, the cuttlefish is related to the squid but has an internal shell known as a cuttlebone. The ink it discharges to distract predators provides the dark brown sepia pigment used by painters, printers, and homeopaths. Cage birds like to eat cuttlebones for their calcium salts.

PARTS USED: Bone, ink.

ACTIVE INGREDIENTS: Calcium phosphate; calcium chloride.

ACTIONS: Neutralizes excess stomach acid; astringent.

MEDICINAL USE: Chinese physicians use cuttlebones for stomach ulcers and indigestion, pruritis (itchy skin), abscesses, sores, wounds, menstrual problems, and leukorrhea (excessive white vaginal discharge). Unani medicine prescribes them internally for kidney stones, indigestion, and nausea, and externally for inflammation and skin diseases, and as a tooth powder. *Sepia*, the homeopathic remedy made from cuttlefish ink, is given for ulcers, warts, incontinence, menopausal and menstrual problems, and detached apathy resulting from shock.

PREPARATIONS: Powder, homeopathic remedies.

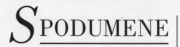

Smilax species, including *S. glabra, S. aristolochiaefolia, S. regelii, S. officinalis, & S. febrifuga*
(Liliaceae) ✔
SARSAPARILLA

Introduced into Europe from Central America in the early 16th century as a cure for syphilis, sarsaparilla was included in many European pharmacopoeias for this use until the 20th century. It is now widely used to flavor medicines and soft drinks. One long established London herbalist, Baldwins, still sells sarsaparilla drinks by the pint. Native to Central America, sarsaparilla is a perennial creeper with a large rhizome and spreading roots. Its thorny stems bear oval leaves with clinging tendrils and clusters of small greenish white flowers.

PARTS USED: Root, rhizome.
ACTIVE INGREDIENTS: Saponins based on smilagin and sarsapogenin, including sarsaponin (pillarin) and smilasaponin; sterols including stigmasterol.
ACTIONS: Stimulates nutrition and elimination; anti-inflammatory; stops itching; relieves gas and colic.
MEDICINAL USE: Given for chronic inflamed skin eruptions such as psoriasis. *S. glabra* and *S. china* are used in Chinese medicine for several conditions, including rheumatism, skin diseases, cystitis, and diarrhea.
PREPARATIONS: Infusion, tablets, tincture, extract.

Smithsonite ⬡
NATIVE ZINC CARBONATE

This mineral has been used since the Middle Ages to produce brass, an alloy of copper and zinc. Zinc is an essential trace element; the existence of communities in Iran and Egypt that have low levels has provided firm evidence of the results of deficiency, which include dwarfism, lack of sexual development, poor hair growth, and rough skin. The way in which zinc works is not fully understood, but it is a component of many enzymes in the body, and is crucial for an effective immune system.

PARTS USED: Zinc oxide or other zinc salts.
ACTIVE INGREDIENTS: Zinc.
ACTIONS: Nutrient; stimulates prostaglandin production; astringent; involved in the formation of new flesh after an injury or operation and in the storage and release of insulin.
MEDICINAL USE: Zinc oxide is applied to the skin in orthodox medicine for rashes, skin eruptions, insect bites, and eczema. Chinese medicine uses smithsonite for the same purposes. Zinc salts (generally zinc sulfate) are given internally as supplements to counteract deficiency and the zinc-lowering effects of certain long-term drug treatments, such as those used to control epilepsy, and of some illnesses, including cystic fibrosis and diabetes. Zinc gluconate is available in preparations for the relief of the common cold.
PREPARATIONS: Powder, over-the-counter lotions, cream, tablets, and capsules.

Solanum dulcamara (Solanaceae) ☠☣
BITTERSWEET, WOODY NIGHTSHADE

Bittersweet is often confused with deadly nightshade (*Atropa belladonna*) by non-botanists; although the two are in the same family, they are entirely different genera. The name bittersweet arose because, on chewing, twigs of solanum taste bitter and then turn sweet. The plant has been used since the time of the ancient Greeks for diverse ailments, including bruises and warts, and sprigs were hung round the necks of sheep to ward off evil spirits. Native to Europe and North America, it is a shrubby trailing perennial with thin woody stems and oval leaves. Deep violet flowers with yellow centers appear during mid- to late summer, followed by red to black berries.

PARTS USED: Two- to three-year-old stems.
ACTIVE INGREDIENTS: Steroidal alkaloids, including soladulcamaridine, solanidine, solasodine, and tomatidine; steroidal saponins, dulcamarin; tannins; resin.
ACTIONS: Anti-inflammatory; antirheumatic; stimulating expectorant; increases bile flow.
MEDICINAL USE: Used in rheumatic disease, psoriasis, and eczema, particularly when the liver is involved, and chronic bronchitis. It is prescribed homeopathically (*Dulcamara*) for a variety of conditions, especially those that come on after getting wet or chilled.
PREPARATIONS: Tincture, homeopathic remedies.

Somniosus microcephalus ⚕
GREENLAND SHARK-HORNED DOGFISH

Until the 19th century, fishermen along the western coasts of Norway and Sweden valued liver oil from the true Greenland shark as a remedy for general debility, irritations of the respiratory and digestive passages, and to speed wound healing. Now, practical trials are confirming these traditional uses. The oils that were identified as active in the shark are now taken from the dogfish *S. microcephalus*. Prevalent in Arctic waters, it is also fished for food and sold as huss or dogfish in fish stores.

PARTS USED: Liver oil.
ACTIVE INGREDIENTS: Alkoxyglycerol fatty acids.
ACTIONS: Tonic.
MEDICINAL USE: Taken before and during radiotherapy treatment for cancer to reduce side effects. It has also been tested as a treatment for cervical cancer and has been shown to improve well-being following treatment and to lengthen survival. The Chinese use it as a general tonic.
PREPARATIONS: Capsules.

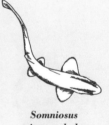

Somniosus microcephalus

Spodumene ⬡
LITHIUM ALUMINUM SILICATE

Found as far and wide as Afghanistan, Brazil, and California, crystals of spodumene can be as long as 18 feet and weigh several tons. The crystals are a source of the mineral lithium, which has not yet been proved to be an essential part of the diet, but is an important medicine for severe mental illness.

PARTS USED: Lithium to make other lithium salts.
ACTIVE INGREDIENTS: Lithium.
ACTIONS: Mood regulating.
MEDICINAL USE: Lithium salts, particularly lithium carbonate, are given in orthodox medicine for manic depression and to control aggressive behavior. Lithium is very toxic, so blood levels of the drugs have to be carefully monitored.
PREPARATIONS: Pharmaceutical preparations.

Stachys betonica/S.officinalis/ Betonica officinalis (Labiatae) 🖋
BETONY, BISHOPSWORT

Betony was so popular in ancient times that it was grown in every monastery and physic garden in Europe. Its reputation is impressive; the Roman emperor Augustus, for example, boasted of its ability to cure at least 47 ailments. Since Egyptian times, it has been thought to possess the ability to dispel evil and was worn about the body to shield "against visions and dreams." Native to Europe, growing best in light sandy soils in sheltered areas, betony is a low-growing perennial herb with square stems, serrated, spear-shaped, rough leaves, and two-lipped, purple flowers in midsummer.

PARTS USED: Whole herb.
ACTIVE INGREDIENTS: Alkaloids, including betonicine, stachydrine, and trigonelline; choline; tannins.
ACTIONS: Promotes wound healing; astringent; circulatory tonic for the brain; relaxing nerve restorative; bitter (digestive stimulant).
MEDICINAL USE: Given internally for nervous headaches, particularly when due to debility, for digestive upsets in nervous states, and in liver and gallbladder disease. It is applied externally as a poultice to heal wounds and bruises.
PREPARATIONS: Infusion, poultice, tincture.

Stellaria media (Caryophyllaceae) 🖋
CHICKWEED, STARWORT, STITCHWORT

A ubiquitous herb that has been known since ancient times, chickweed always grows in close association with human settlements. It is a feed for birds, as well as for all herbivorous animals, who relish it, and has also been used as a vegetable. Native to Europe, chickweed is now so widespread that it is naturalized on farmland as well as wasteland, especially in urban areas. This delicate annual herb spreads vigorously, sending out many branched, delicate stems. It has small, oval, bright, pale green leaves and white starlike flowers all summer.

PARTS USED: Whole herb.
ACTIVE INGREDIENTS: PARTS USED: Saponins; coumarins; flavonoids; triterpenoids; carboxylic acids; vitamin C.

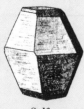

Sulfur

ACTIONS: Stops itching; promotes wound healing; soothes and softens skin; astringent.
MEDICINAL USE: Applied externally to soothe itchy and inflamed skin diseases such as eczema and related dermatitis. It is also used as a poultice on skin eruptions and taken internally for rheumatic diseases. *S. alsine* is prescribed in Chinese medicine for colds, snakebites, spots, and traumatic injuries.
PREPARATIONS: Poultice, cream, tincture.

Succinum 🎲
AMBER

The fossilized gum of fir trees that lived up to 300 million years ago, amber has the property of taking on a small electric charge when rubbed, and can then pick up light objects. This led to the use of the Greek word for amber, *elektron*, to form the term electricity. Honey yellow or reddish brown, amber has always been sought after as a gemstone, the most valuable amber coming from around the Baltic Sea. And, it will float on water and burn, like the wood it came from.

PARTS USED: Amber stone.
ACTIVE INGREDIENTS: Succoxyabietic; succinosilvic and succinoabietinolic acids.
ACTIONS: Sedative; increases urine production; stimulates menstruation; anti-infective.
MEDICINAL USE: Chinese physicians prescribe it for insomnia, anxiety, forgetfulness, nervous seizures, for urinary retention or painful urination, to encourage menstruation, to reduce swelling, and to speed healing.
PREPARATIONS: Ground.

Sulfur 🎲

The yellow to brown crystals of sulfur have been used in medicine for at least 4,000 years. This was long before it was known that every cell in the human body contains sulfur, as do all plant and animal cells. In man, the mineral is concentrated in hair, nails, and skin. There is no recommended daily intake of sulfur because it is so widespread in food that deficiency is unlikely. However, in the past, generations of Western children were given extra sulfur, in the form of brimstone and treacle, to "cleanse the blood."

PARTS USED: Sulfur.
ACTIVE INGREDIENTS: Sulfur.
ACTIONS: Laxative; mild antiseptic.
MEDICINAL USE: Applied externally in Western and Chinese medicine for scabies, acne, dandruff, and other skin problems. Chinese medicine uses it internally for lower back pain, kidney "chills," constipation, and impotence. Given in homeopathic medicine (*Sulfur*) for skin problems, diarrhea, body odor, oversweating, lack of stamina, and oversensitivity to the cold.
PREPARATIONS: Cream, ointment, lotion, powder, paste, pills, homeopathic remedies.

Symphytum officinale (Boraginaceae) ✎
COMFREY, HEALING HERB, BONESET

A plant high in protein, comfrey is used as an animal feed and organic manure as well as a medicine. The name boneset derives from its useful property of healing broken bones and wounds; it has even been used by orthopedic surgeons on complicated bone fractures. This property has been known at least since Roman times, when it was named *conferva*, meaning to join together. Recently there has been concern that the pyrrolizidine alkaloids contained in comfrey may damage the liver. However, this has been shown only with high doses of plant extracts and not with normal therapeutic doses of whole herb. A native of Europe and Asia, comfrey thrives on moist or wet wasteland and meadows. It is a perennial with a deep black root, bristly green stems, and large, succulent, hairy leaves. White, pink, or purple, bell-shaped flowers are produced throughout the spring and summer.

PARTS USED: Whole herb, root.
ACTIVE INGREDIENTS: Allantoin; pyrrolizidine alkaloids; phenolic acids, including rosmarinic, chlorogenic, and caffeic; mucilage; choline; tannins; saponins.
ACTIONS: Soothes internal body surfaces; promotes wound healing; stimulates bone, connective tissue, and cartilage repair; soothing astringent; relaxing expectorant.
MEDICINAL USE: Used externally as a healing agent on wounds, ulcers, fractures, and sprains and strains of muscles and joints. It is given internally for stomach ulcers and erosions, colitis (inflammation of the intestines), and bronchitis.
PREPARATIONS: Dried herb and root, cream, tincture.
CAUTION: **Because of concern about the pyrrolizidine alkaloids, internal treatment should be restricted to a few weeks only; external application need not be restricted.**

Syzigium aromaticum/Eugenia aromatica (Myrtaceae) ✎
CLOVES

Cloves are the dried flower buds of the tree. They were used in the Far East as a ceremonial herb and a medicine for centuries before they reached Europe in the 4th century. The trees are native to the Moluccas in the East Indies but have since been introduced to other tropical islands for commercial production. An evergreen tree, *S. aromaticum* has undulating, bright green, spear-shaped leaves with a strong scent and clusters of yellow flowers in summer, which turn into small berries.

PARTS USED: Oil from flower buds.
ACTIVE INGREDIENTS: Volatile oil containing eugenol, methyl salicylate, and sesquiterpenes; flavonoids kaempferol and rhamnetin; sterols, including sitosterol, campesterol, and stigmasterol.
ACTIONS: Stimulant; eases pain; relieves gas and colic; aromatic.
MEDICINAL USE: Widely used externally to relieve toothache. Internally, it is given for stomach infections with indigestion, and has been used to treat worms.
PREPARATIONS: Clove water, oil.

Tanacetum parthenium/ Chrysanthemum parthenium (Compositae) ✎
FEVERFEW, FEATHERFEW

Folk medicine used this herb for many conditions; today feverfew's benefits in relieving headaches, uterus problems, and general aches and pains have led to a resurgence in its use. Feverfew is also an effective insect repellent. It is native to southern Europe but is widely spread throughout the world. A perennial, it has a mass of bright, yellowish green, slightly hairy, pointed leaves, which look almost fernlike and have a pungent odor. Its flat, daisylike flowers grow throughout the summer months.

PARTS USED: Whole herb.
ACTIVE INGREDIENTS: Volatile oil containing pinene and bornyl acetate; sesquiterpene lactones, including parthenolide; chrysanthemonin; acetylene derivatives.
ACTIONS: Reduces or prevents fever; dilates the blood vessels; relieves pain; kills and helps expel worms; stimulates the stomach; antirheumatic.
MEDICINAL USE: Given for migraine headaches, arthritis, menstrual cramps, and after birth to help restore the uterus. Although chewing fresh leaves is recommended for headaches, some people may develop mouth ulcers and it may be preferable to crush the leaves and eat them between two slices of bread.
PREPARATIONS: Fresh leaves, powdered leaves, tablets, tincture.

Taraxacum officinalis (Compositae) ✎
DANDELION, LION'S TOOTH, PRIEST'S CROWN

Dandelion is one of most useful and common European herbs. Its leaves provide a safe and effective diuretic, and have been compared favorably with the common pharmaceutical drug furosemide. Its root is an excellent tonic herb for liver and gallbladder problems. Although dandelion was introduced into European medicine only in the 16th century, its reputation as a medicine grew as it became a popular salad herb and coffee substitute. A native to Europe and Asia, it is now found in open, sunny places throughout the world. Dandelion has a strong deep taproot that supports a rosette of spear-shaped, serrated, hairy leaves and yellow daisylike flowers which appear from early spring and close up at night and in overcast weather.

PARTS USED: Root and leaves.
ACTIVE INGREDIENTS: Sesquiterpene lactones; bitter principle, taraxacin; triterpenes including taraxol,

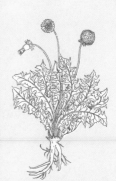

Taraxacum officinalis

taraxerol, and stigmasterol; phenolic acids; polysaccharides; carotenoids.

ACTIONS: Increases urine production; tonic; antirheumatic; laxative; increases the flow of bile.

MEDICINAL USE: Given internally as a liver tonic and remedy for gallbladder inflammation due to gallstones and for jaundice. It is also used as a diuretic for raised blood pressure and water retention, as a laxative where liver problems and indigestion are involved, as a useful adjunct in the treatment of toxic conditions causing skin disease, and for rheumatic conditions. Fresh juice is applied directly to warts. Chinese medicine prescribes dandelion for boils and abscesses, stomachache, and breast problems.

PREPARATIONS: Fresh, dried, infusion, decoction of root, tincture.

Thymus vulgaris & T. serpyllum
(Labiatae)
GARDEN THYME; LEMON THYME

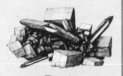

Titanite

Both a common culinary herb and one of the most useful household medicines, thyme was known in ancient Rome as the source of the best honey in Athens and was often used as an insecticide by burning the leaves. Throughout history it has been used for coughs, lung infections, and stomach complaints, and in the 18th century the volatile oil thymol was isolated and discovered to be one of the most powerful natural antiseptics. Native to the mountains of southern Europe, thyme is a creeping aromatic perennial with thin wiry stems and small, oblong, succulent leaves. Its flowers appear in early summer as clusters of small, pinkish blooms.

PARTS USED: Whole herb, collected in flower.

ACTIVE INGREDIENTS: Volatile oil containing thymol, carvacrol, cineole, borneol, linalool, and pinene; flavonoids apigenin and luteolin; tannins.

ACTIONS: Antiseptic; expectorant; relieves gas and colic; reduces muscle tension and spasms.

MEDICINAL USE: Used as an expectorant for whooping cough, bronchitis, and congested lungs, as a gargle for throat and mouth infections, and to help settle indigestion and flatulence. It can be applied as a disinfectant and to heal wounds.

PREPARATIONS: Infusion, oil, tincture.

Tilia x europea (Tiliaceae)
SMALL-LEAVED EUROPEAN LINDEN

American scientists recently found that children with flu recovered more quickly and with fewer complications on tilia tea than with antibiotics. This bears out the traditional use in Europe of tilia tisanes for colds and "fevers." It is, in fact, the most popular daily tisane in France, where its gentle relaxing properties are employed to help parents cope with irritable children. American linden, *T. americana*, has similar uses. Native to Europe, *T. x europea* grows in woodland, and is an ornamental plant on footpaths and in parks. A tall, deciduous tree, it has a smooth bark, white wood, toothed, heart-shaped leaves, and sweet smelling flowers in spring.

PARTS USED: Flowers.

ACTIVE INGREDIENTS: Volatile oil containing farnesol; flavonoids, including hesperidin, quercetin, and astralagin; mucilage; tannins.

ACTIONS: Restores the nerves; reduces muscle tension and spasms; controls low blood pressure; induces sweating.

MEDICINAL USE: Given as a gentle relaxant to relieve anxiety and irritability, and nervous states that affect digestion, blood pressure, and bowel function. It is also used for fevers, colds, and flu.

PREPARATIONS: Infusion, tincture.

Titanite
CALCIUM TITANIUM SILICATE

Titanite is the main source of titanium, which is a jewelry metal and a protective ingredient in suntan products. Its combination of lightness and great strength makes titanium an important metal in spacecraft and high-speed aircraft. Titanite itself is also sometimes cut and polished for use as a jewel stone.

PARTS USED: Titanium to make titanium dioxide.

ACTIVE INGREDIENTS: Titanium.

ACTIONS: Absorbs ultraviolet light.

MEDICINAL USE: Applied externally to shield the skin from ultraviolet rays and prevent sunburn, and to soothe the skin in inflammatory skin conditions such as eczema.

PREPARATIONS: Over-the-counter suntan products, cream.

Trifolium pratense (Leguminosae)
RED CLOVER, TREFOIL

Although a native European plant, it was not until clover was naturalized in North America and Native Americans had discovered its medicinal properties that it was recognized as a medicine in Europe. It is reputed to be a valuable external remedy for the treatment of cancers, but this has not been proven. A perennial with hairy stems and leaves of three spear-shaped leaflets, it produces red to purple flowers in the summer.

PARTS USED: Flowers.

ACTIVE INGREDIENTS: Isoflavones; flavonoids; coumarins.

ACTIONS: Stimulates nutrition and elimination; dermatological agent; reduces muscle tension and spasms; expectorant.

MEDICINAL USE: Commonly used for skin diseases, including eczema and psoraisis. Also sometimes included in cough mixtures.

PREPARATIONS: Infusion, tincture.

Tropaeolum majus (Tropaeolaceae)
NASTURTIUM, INDIAN CRESS

The Spanish conquistadors brought seeds of nasturtium back to Europe from South America after rampaging through Peru in the 16th century. The leaves are eaten in salad for their piquancy and the seeds are used as a cheap substitute for capers. An annual creeping plant with weak succulent stems and lobed leaves, it typically produces red flowers but there are also hybrids with flowers of orange and shades of yellow.

PARTS USED: Whole herb.
ACTIVE INGREDIENTS: Volatile oil; glycoside, glucotropaeoline.
ACTIONS: Antibiotic.
MEDICINAL USE: Used internally for infections of the urinary tract and respiratory system. It is also applied externally as an antiseptic to wounds and skin eruptions.
PREPARATIONS: Fresh leaves, tincture.

Tussilago farfara (Compositae)
COLTSFOOT, HORSEHOOF, COUGHWORT, BRITISH TOBACCO

This plant was originally recorded as leafless because the flowers appear directly from the ground and wither days or weeks before the first leaf emerges from the soil. It has been considered one of the best herbs for coughs since the time of the classical authorities Pliny and Dioscorides, as reflected in the common name coughwort. Today, it is believed that smoking the leaves of coltsfoot benefits asthma and bronchitis sufferers. Native to Europe and thriving on moist wasteland, it is a perennial with creeping stems and yellow daisylike flowers in early spring. Large, downy, hoof-shaped leaves are produced after flowering.

PARTS USED: Leaves, flowers.
ACTIVE INGREDIENTS: Flavonoids, including rutin, hyperoside, and isoquercetin; pyrrolizidine alkaloids; mucilage; tannins.
ACTIONS: Inhibits coughing; expectorant; soothes internal body surfaces; anti-inflammatory; promotes wound healing locally.
MEDICINAL USE: Given to soothe dry irritable, coughs, especially those with a nervous component. It is also thought helpful in reducing the bronchial spasms of asthma and bronchitis.
PREPARATIONS: Infusion, syrup, tobacco, tincture.

Ulmus rubra/U. fulva (Ulmaceae)
SLIPPERY ELM, RED ELM, INDIAN ELM

This North American tree was used by Native Americans as a treatment for constipation because of the copious mucilage it contains, and for diarrhea because of its astringency. Once adopted as a European medicine, it was also used as a nutritive and as a poultice. Only the inner bark of slippery elm is used, the harvest of which usually kills the tree. Found in poor soils along the East Coast of the United States, this tree has a rough bark and oval, serrated leaves. Its flowers are tiny, grow in clusters, and produce small seeds surrounded by a circular papery "wing."

PARTS USED: Inner bark.
ACTIVE INGREDIENTS: Mucilage; tannins.
ACTIONS: Soothes internal body surfaces; softens and soothes the skin; nutritive.
MEDICINAL USE: Given to soothe sore throats and inflammation of the lining of the digestive tract. Also used in debility as a source of energy, and applied as a poultice on boils, abscesses, and infected wounds.
PREPARATIONS: Powder, tablets, poultice.

Urtica dioica (Urticaceae)
STINGING NETTLE

The Romans used to flail their rheumatic joints with nettles and rub the leaves on their bodies to warm them up in British winters. The sting, which is due to ammonia in special hairs on the leaves, stimulates blood circulation. Drying or heating the leaves deactivates this stinging chemical. Nettle also contains vitamin C and iron, and increases the absorption of the latter. A native of Europe and Asia but naturalized throughout the world, it has heart-shaped leaves with normal and stinging hairs, and flowers throughout summer.

PARTS USED: Whole herb.
ACTIVE INGREDIENTS: Indoles, including histamine and serotonin; formic acid; acetylcholine; vitamins A and C; minerals, including iron, silica, and potassium.
ACTIONS: Prevents hemorrhage; circulatory stimulant; dermatological agent; stimulates milk production; mildly lowers blood sugar levels.
MEDICINAL USE: The juice of nettle is used for skin conditions and rheumatism. Nettle is also given as a tonic in anemia, for non-insulin-dependent diabetes, and to help lactating mothers maintain their milk supply. A related species, *U. urens*, is prescribed in homeopathy for rheumatic pains, burns, and nettle rash.
PREPARATIONS: Juice, fresh herb, infusions, tincture, homeopathic remedies.

Valeriana officinalis (Valerianaceae)
VALERIAN, ALL-HEAL, GARDEN HELIOTROPE

Cats are driven into a euphoric frenzy by the smell of valerian root, while the human response is one of sedation and relaxation. In traditional medicine, it was so revered that it was called all-heal and, during the Second World War, both shell shock and "bombing neurosis" were treated with valerian. The distinctive smell of the herb, which is absent from the fresh plant, arises when the roots are dried. Native to Europe and west Asia but now naturalized in North America, it grows in low-lying sandy meadows and near streams. It is a perennial with a conical rhizome, thick roots, and compound leaves made up of spearlike segments. Small pink to white flowers appear in midsummer, which produce tiny downy seeds that are carried on the wind.

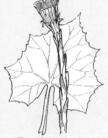

Tussilago farfara

PARTS USED: Root.

ACTIVE INGREDIENTS: Volatile oil containing valerenic, isovalerenic, and isovaleric acids as a result of the hydrolysis of the valepotriates; iridoid esters known as valepotriates; alkaloids,. including actinidine, valerine, valerianine, and chatinine; flavonoids; tannins.

ACTIONS: Sedative; promotes sleep; reduces muscle tension and spasms; lowers blood pressure; mildly increases urine production; expectorant.

MEDICINAL USE: Used internally for anxiety, insomnia, nervous tension, and irritable bowel syndrome, and applied locally for muscle spasms and cramping. Chinese physicians prescribe it for flu, rheumatism, insomnia, apprehension, and traumatic injuries.

PREPARATIONS: Tablets, tincture.

Viburnum opulus & V. prunifolium
(Caprifoliaceae) ✿

CRAMP BARK, GUELDER ROSE, EUROPEAN CRANBERRY BUSH; NANNYBERRY, BLACK HAW

Chaucer knew the medicinal benefits of this plant, which grows wild in hedgerows throughout Britain; he advised that one should "picke hem right as they grow and ete hem in." The European species (*V. opulus*) has similar constituents and uses to the American (*V. prunifolium*) and both are often combined in prescriptions. Native to Europe, North Africa, and western Asia, *V. opulus* is a small shrub with lobed leaves and clusters of small white flowers which appear in midsummer and are followed by bunches of red and scarlet edible berries.

PARTS USED: Bark.

ACTIVE INGREDIENTS: Hydroquinnones, including arbutin and hydroquinnone; coumarins, including scopoletin and scopoline; tannins.

ACTIONS: Reduces muscle tension and spasms; sedative; astringent.

MEDICINAL USE: Given to relieve menstrual cramps and general muscle cramping, particularly of the intestine. It is also useful in the treatment of threatened miscarriage.

PREPARATIONS: Decoction, tincture.

Vinca major & V. minor
(Apocynaceae) ✿

GREATER PERIWINKLE; LESSER PERIWINKLE

A plant rich in superstitious legends, greater periwinkle has been said to induce love between a man and his wife if eaten in a mixture of earthworms and houseleek. In addition, however, it has been associated with death and placed on the coffins of children. A native of Europe, thriving on alkaline soils, *V. major* is a perennial creeper with purple five-petalled flowers in early summer and glossy oval leaves.

PARTS USED: Whole herb.

ACTIVE INGREDIENTS: Indole alkaloids, including majdine, majordine, akuammigine, reserpine, sarpagine, serpentine, and vincamajine; tannins.

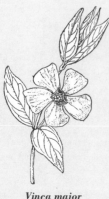

Vinca major

ACTIONS: Prevents hemorrhage; astringent.

MEDICINAL USE: Used internally to treat excess menstrual bleeding and vaginal discharges, and externally to treat nosebleeds and hemorrhoids. *V. minor* is used in homeopathy (*Vinca*) for hemorrhages. The related plant *Catharanthus roseus* is the source of two alkaloid drugs, vincristine and vinblastine, which are used in the treatment of leukemia and Hodgkin's disease in orthodox medicine.

PREPARATIONS: Infusion, tincture, homeopathic remedies.

Viola tricolor (Violaceae) ✿
HEARTSEASE, EUROPEAN WILD PANSY

This is a traditional remedy for mending broken hearts (but not for heart disease), which is reflected in its many regional names. It has been used for centuries to treat inflammatory skin conditions and against scabs and itchings of the whole body. A native of Europe, it is a short annual or biennial herb with fragile stems and spear-shaped serrated leaves. Yellow, white, and purple flowers in the classic pansy shape appear throughout the summer.

PARTS USED: Whole herb.

ACTIVE INGREDIENTS: Flavonoids; saponins; methyl salicylate; resin; tannins.

ACTIONS: Anti-inflammatory; increases urine production; antirheumatic; expectorant.

MEDICINAL USE: Given to treat skin disease, particularly eczema, and for rheumatism, gout, and chronic bronchitis.

PREPARATIONS: Infusion, tincture.

Viscum album (Loranthaceae) ✿
MISTLETOE

Mistletoe is a true parasite, which may explain the strong magical associations that the plant attracted, and which are still evident in the custom of hanging it in houses at Christmas. For the ancient druids it was sacred, and sprigs were held to dispel evil spirits. The Latin name *Viscum* refers to the stickiness of the seeds, a property essential to the propagation of mistletoe, as its seed must stick to the trunk of its host long enough to germinate and insert a specialized root into the bark for nutrients. Native to Europe, mistletoe has evergreen, leathery, oar-shaped leaves and tiny flowers in early summer, followed by pale green to white berries that ripen in late autumn.

PARTS USED: Leaves, berries.

ACTIVE INGREDIENTS: Glycoproteins; viscotoxins; phenolic acids; flavonoids; lignans.

ACTIONS Dilates the blood vessels; lowers blood pressure; sedative; reputedly anticancer.

MEDICINAL USE: Given for high blood pressure associated with arterial disease, particularly when nervous conditions are present.

PREPARATIONS: Decoction, tincture, tablets.

CAUTION: **Use only under the guidance of a qualified practitioner.**

Vitex agnus-castus (Verbenaceae)
CHASTEBERRY, CHASTE TREE, HEMP TREE, MONK'S PEPPER

Chasteberry is reputed to reduce the sex urge of men and to help with female hormonal imbalances. In the past, celibate monks turned to this herb, as did Greek women who wanted no more additions to their family, giving it to their menfolk. Even now, its flowers are cast on the floor when male novices enter Italian monasteries for the first time. A native of the Mediterranean, it is a perennial shrub with palm-shaped leaves and small purple flowers in the summer, which are followed by tiny seeds. The whole plant is strongly aromatic.

PARTS USED: Seeds.
ACTIVE INGREDIENTS: Iridoid glycosides, including aucibin and agnuside; volatile oil; fixed oil; flavonoids, including casticin.
ACTIONS: Hormonal, it acts on the pituitary gland in the brain, stimulating the release of lutenizing hormone, which stimulates progesterone production.
MEDICINAL USE: Used to treat premenstrual syndrome, excessive menstrual flow, and menopausal symptoms.
PREPARATIONS: Infusion, tincture.

Zanthoxylum americanum (Rutaceae)
PRICKLY ASH, TOOTHBRUSH BUSH

Native Americans used prickly ash to cure the excruciating pain of toothache. It was brought to Europe in the mid-19th century for the same purpose but is now also a recognized circulatory stimulant and has a wide application in natural medicine. Found only in the United States on rich woodland soil, it is a shrub with palm-shaped leaves and sharp spines on its branches. Flowers appear in early spring.

PARTS USED: Bark, berries.
ACTIVE INGREDIENTS: Quaternary alkaloids, including chelerythrine, magnoflorine, nitidine, and laurifoline; pyranocoumarins, including xanthyletin and xanthoxyletin; volatile oil.
ACTIONS: Circulatory stimulant; local counter-irritant; induces sweating; antirheumatic; promotes saliva production.
MEDICINAL USE: Used to treat skin, joint, and general inflammatory disorders when sluggish circulation is a factor, and for debilitated digestion associated with colic and flatulence. In Chinese medicine, prickly ash is prescribed for very similar conditions.
PREPARATIONS: Decoction, tincture, tablets.

Zea mays (Graminae)
CORN, MAIZE, INDIAN CORN

Corn is a valuable cereal; the kernels have fibrous coats that help relieve constipation, and contain starch, protein, and an oil rich in polyunsaturated fatty acids, which lower the risk of heart disease. In addition, the silks, which are usually discarded when corn-on-the-cob is eaten, are prized as a herb for common urinary tract ailments. Native to South America but now cultivated throughout the world, it is an annual grass, with male and female flowers on each plant. As soon as the ovaries in the cob are fertilized, the stigmas dry to a rusty brown and the yellow kernels develop.

PARTS USED: Stigmas, styles.
ACTIVE INGREDIENTS: Saponins; allantoin; sterols and stigmasterol; alkaloid, hordenine; polyphenols.
ACTIONS: Increases urine production; soothes internal body surfaces.
MEDICINAL USE: Used for inflammatory conditions of the urinary tract such as cystitis, bladder and kidney infections, and kidney stones.
PREPARATIONS: Infusion, tincture.

Zingiber officinalis (Zingiberaceae)
GINGER

Ginger is often thought of as being an Oriental spice, but the ancient Greeks used ginger as medicine too and the Romans had ginger in their medicinal supplies when they invaded Britain in 43 AD. Native to Southeast Asia, it has been introduced worldwide in the tropics, where it is often grown commercially; the best quality ginger now comes from Jamaica. The Chinese regard ginger so highly that they include it as an ingredient in about half of all prescriptions. It is a perennial with a thick tuberous root, long tapering leaves, and purplish flowers in spikes. The roots are harvested after the leaves have died during the autumn.

PARTS USED: Root.
ACTIVE INGREDIENTS: Volatile oil containing cineole, borneol, zingiberene, camphene, citral, bisabolene, and beta-phellandrene; resinous matter containing gingerols, gingerdiols, zingerone, and shogoals.
ACTIONS: Circulatory stimulant; relieves gas and colic; induces sweating; lowers blood cholesterol levels; prevents motion sickness.
MEDICINAL USE: Given for poor peripheral (local) circulation causing cold limbs and as a warming circulatory stimulant in lung infections. It is also used to prevent motion sickness, and for indigestion and flatulence. Widely prescribed in Chinese medicine for similar uses and for diarrhea, general lack of energy, coughs, and colds. Tablets of ginger are available over-the-counter for motion sickness.
PREPARATIONS: Fresh root, infusion, tincture, powder, over-the-counter tablets.

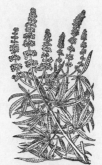

Vitex agnus-castus

Home Remedies

MOST HOMES have a medicine cabinet filled with pharmaceutical drugs that have accumulated over the years. These drugs come in many forms, such as tablets and capsules, creams and ointments, syrups and other liquids, powders, suppositories, pessaries, and sprays. Each is designed to deliver its active ingredient to where it is needed in the body in the most effective way.

The preparation of natural remedies is approached in the same way. The healing powers of natural material can be released only if the material is prepared in the correct manner to ensure that as many of the active ingredients are extracted as possible, and that they are made available to the body in the most convenient form. When preparing a herbal remedy, for example, the particular part of the plant containing the active ingredients must be harvested and stored to preserve its constituents. Then, the active ingredients have to be extracted and prepared in the most appropriate way for the healing task.

Natural remedies are available from health food stores, herbalists, pharmacists, and specialist manufacturers, but some can also be made in the home if the simple guidelines outlined here are followed. Although a qualified practitioner is the best person to decide what remedy to use, and when and how much, the medicine kit overleaf explains how simple preparations of a small number of readily available and safe herbs can be used in the treatment of common ailments.

Harvesting herbs

Many of the most useful medicinal plants can be harvested, dried, and stored for home use. Before harvesting a herb, be absolutely certain of its identity. This is not so much to avoid confusing poisonous with less poisonous plants, but to avoid mistaking closely related species that may contain different active ingredients. Always collect specimen leaves, flowers, fruit, and bark to check the identity of all unfamiliar plants.

Next, check which part of the herb is required, such as the whole herb, flowers, fruit, leaves, stems, or root. The wrong part of the right plant may have no medicinal value. Also be sure to pick good quality material at the prime time. Most herbs are best harvested during their flowering period.

Once you have harvested a herb, preserve the material carefully to avoid loss of its essential activity. Spread the material out to dry soon after it has been harvested; drying inactivates any enzymes and prevents natural chemical reactions in plant material which would otherwise alter the active ingredients present. However, do not dry plants containing volatile oils, such as lemon balm (*Melissa officinalis*), peppermint (*Mentha* x *piperita*), or German chamomile (*Matricaria recutita*), in the sun or indoors above 100°F, as heat can cause the oils to evaporate. Roots or bark, however, can be dried in the sun, but are best placed on racks or spread out on newspaper in a warm, dry, shady place.

When the material has dried, store it in cardboard boxes or paper bags, not in glass jars or plastic bags, which can encourage the growth of damaging mold. Store the boxes or bags in a dark, dry room that is well-ventilated.

Labelling herbs

Once dried, most herbs look the same to the inexpert eye, so clearly label any plant material collected with the name and date; the date is important so that old material can be discarded. Dried herbs can be bought, but be fussy about the choice of supplier and make sure the herbs are clearly and accurately labelled. Check the date of harvesting and the method of both drying and storage. If treated carefully, dried herbs should retain their quality for at least 12 months.

Herbal recipes

The choice of preparation is decided normally by the type of active ingredients in an herb and the purpose of the medicine. Liquid preparations such as infusions or tinctures are used internally either to treat problems of the digestive and upper respiratory tracts directly or to carry medicines to the stomach for absorption and circulation around the body. They are also used externally, for example as douches.

Creams and ointments deliver healing agents to the skin or to structures such as muscles and joints that lie just beneath it. Poultices and compresses also direct remedies to particular areas of the skin.

Powdered herbs may be taken as snuff to deliver a medicine to the membranes of the nose, while inhalations of volatile oils carry medicines straight to the delicate tissues deep in the lungs. Pessaries and suppositories are efficient ways of placing medicines in the vagina and rectum for absorption.

Preparations such as tinctures and creams are even more easily confused than dried herbs. Avoid confusion by ensuring careful labelling at all stages of remedy preparation and storage.

Infusions

The simplest way to take a remedy is as an infusion. Infusions are used when plant material is easily penetrated by water and its active ingredients dissolve readily in hot water. Most leaves and flowers are suitable for use in infusions, roots and barks less so.

Standard recipe. Infusions are made by steeping herbs in boiling water for at least 15 minutes in a pot with a close-fitting lid (an ordinary teapot is suitable). The use of a lid is particularly important when making an infusion with an herb containing volatile oils, so that when the oils vaporize with the steam, they condense on the lid and drip back into the infusion.

1 ounce finely chopped dried material
1 pint boiling water
STANDARD DOSE: $3/4$ of a cup taken three times a day

Allow the mixture to stand in the pot for at least 15 minutes and then strain off the infused liquid. If all the infusion is not to be used immediately, let it cool in the pot before straining it off. Store infusions in the refrigerator and use within 24 hours. When instructions refer to a fresh infusion, they mean one freshly made, not one made from freshly harvested material.

———— • ————

Decoctions
Bark, stems, and roots of herbs are not only usually thicker than leaves but also contain a substance called lignan which is difficult to dissolve in water. The decoction process is a more vigorous extraction than that for infusions. Roots of marsh mallow (*Althaea officinalis*) and dandelion (*Taraxacum officinalis*) are typically made into decoctions.

Standard recipe. Decoctions are prepared by boiling chopped or finely divided material in a saucepan of water for 10–20 minutes. It is optional to soak the material first in water for 12 hours.

1 ounce chopped or finely divided material
1 pint water
STANDARD DOSE: $3/4$ of a cup taken three times a day

As the mixture boils, some water evaporates. So, once the liquid has been strained off, top it off to the original 1 pint with more water. Store decoctions in the refrigerator and use within 24 hours.

Tinctures
Tinctures are prepared with solvents such as alcohol or glycerol to extract constituents that are either insoluble or only partially soluble in water. Alcohol is the most common solvent and can be used in strengths of 45, 60, 70, and 90 percent. Substances such as the resins in myrrh (*Commiphora molmol*) or calendula (*Calendula officinalis*) are more soluble in the higher percentage alcohols but 45 percent is the most commonly used strength. Tinctures also have the advantage of preserving extracted ingredients for 12 months or more.

Standard recipe. Simple tinctures can be made at home using vodka or Polish spirit of at least 60 proof (30 percent alcohol). Lower strengths of alcohol do extract useful amounts of active ingredients but are not preservative. Usually, a 1:5 tincture (as below) is prepared.

3 ounces finely chopped or ground dried material
15 fluid ounces alcohol
STANDARD DOSE: one 5ml spoonful taken three times a day

Mix the ingredients in a wide-mouthed sealable jar, and place this in the dark. Shake the mixture daily for two weeks, then strain off the tincture into an opaque bottle for storage. In practice, there are wide variations in recommended tincture dosages, depending on the remedy being used, the age of the patient, and the condition being treated.

———— • ————

Syrups
Syrups are often used both as a way of preserving extracted ingredients, and as an effective method of giving soothing cough or throat medicines like wild cherry (*Prunus serotina*), marsh mallow (*Althaea officinalis*), and licorice (*Glycyrrhiza glabra*).

Standard recipe. Syrups are made by mixing sugar with an infusion or decoction, or by adding a tincture to a solution of sugar and water.

Two parts by weight of white cane sugar to one part decoction, infusion, or water; the water/sugar solution to be added three parts by volume to one part tincture
STANDARD DOSE: three 5ml spoonfuls sipped every 3 hours

Creams and ointments
Creams are a mixture of a medicine and an oily base that is designed to hold the remedy in place for external use. Creams are light and slightly oily, thus allowing them to merge with the skin's secretions so that the active ingredients they contain can penetrate the skin. Ointments tend to be heavier and oilier than creams. They are designed so that they do not merge with the skin's secretions and are used to apply protective remedies, such as emollients, to the surface of the skin.

Standard recipe. A simple and soothing skin cream can be made by combining a tincture or infusion with a mixture of almond oil, beeswax, and lanolin.

1 cup almond oil
4 ounces white beeswax
4 ounces anhydrous lanolin
1 cup tincture, or
2 cups fresh infusion

Place the almond oil, beeswax, and lanolin in the top of a double boiler until they have melted. Heat the tincture or infusion to the same temperature and add it to the double boiler. Heat this mixture until it is just simmering and all the water has boiled off. Remove it from the heat immediately and before the oil overheats; this can damage the herbal extracts now absorbed within the mixture. After allowing the mixture to cool until it is lukewarm, pour it into clean, screw-top, glass jars for setting and storage. Creams will keep for 6 months in a cool dark place.

———— • ————

Plasters, compresses, and poultices
These preparations offer methods of applying remedies directly to the skin. Plasters and compresses are made of cotton bandages soaked in infusion or decoction and wrapped around the affected area or held on with pressure. Compresses are also warm. Poultices are moistened herbs placed on the skin and held there with a bandage. Moistened and warmed herbal tea bags also make excellent poultices. Tea bags of chamomile, for example, can be applied to help soothe and heal insect bites and eczema.

Natural Medicine Kit

A wide range of mishaps and ailments can be quickly and effectively relieved with natural medicines. Furthermore, unlike pharmaceutical preparations, many natural remedies are ready for use in the form in which they are found. This section describes a kit of common remedies and lists everyday ailments they can be used to treat. It is often difficult for the layperson to decide when symptoms are serious enough to require professional intervention. It is important to remember that symptoms such as fevers, abdominal pains, fainting spells, or headaches can indicate serious disease. If you are in any doubt, or if your symptoms persist for more than three days, it is important to seek advice from a qualified practitioner.

Remedy Guide for Self-treatment

Remedy symbols: ⌀ = cream ✔ = fresh leaves ✿ = homeopathic tablets (see p. 24 for explanation of x strengths) ☕ = infusion ⬤ = decoction ⚘ = poultice ✕ = tincture

AILMENT	REMEDY	DOSAGE	AILMENT	REMEDY	DOSAGE
Acne	calendula ✕	2 – 3x daily	Cuts and abrasions	calendula ⚘ ✕	2 – 3x daily
Athlete's foot	calendula ⬤ ✕ ⌀	2 – 3x daily		chamomile ⚘ ⬤	2 – 3x daily
	thyme ⬤ ✕	2 – 3x daily		garlic, crushed	2 – 3x daily
Blood pressure, high	linden ⬤	3x daily		plantain ⚘	2 – 3x daily
			Cystitis	plantain ⬤	3x daily
Boils	calendula ⚘ ✕	2 – 3x daily		thyme ⬤	3x daily
	garlic, crushed	2 – 3x daily	Earache, catarrhal	elder ⬤	3x daily
Breasts, swollen	dandelion ✔	10 – 15 daily	Eczema	calendula ⌀ ⬤	2 – 3x daily
	dandelion ⬤	3x daily		chamomile ⚘	2 – 3x daily
	dandelion ✕	3x daily	Edema	dandelion ✔	10 – 15 daily
Bronchitis	elder ⬤	3x daily		dandelion ⬤	3x daily
	garlic, fresh	3 – 5 cloves daily		dandelion ✕	3x daily
	thyme ⬤	3x daily	Eye infections (including conjunctivitis)	calendula ⬤	As an eyewash 2 – 3x daily
	thyme ✕	3x daily		elder ⬤	As an eyewash 2 – 3x daily
Bruises	arnica ✿	6 or 12x every 2 hours for 6 doses	Flatulence	chamomile ⬤	3x daily
	arnica ⌀	2 – 3x daily		chamomile ✕	3x daily
Burns, minor	calendula ⌀	2 – 3x daily		ginger ⬤	3x daily
	elder ⬤	2 – 3x daily		lemon balm ⬤	3x daily
Chilblains	ginger ⬤	3x daily	Flu	elder ⬤	3x daily
Cold hands/feet	ginger ⬤	3x daily		linden ⬤	3x daily
Cold sores	lemon balm ✕	2 – 3x daily	Food poisoning	garlic, fresh	3 – 5 cloves daily
Colds	elder ⬤	3x daily		thyme ⬤	3x daily
	garlic, fresh	3 – 5 cloves daily	Fungal infections	calendula ⬤	As a douche 2 – 3x daily
	ginger ⬤	3x daily		chamomile ⬤	As a douche 2 – 3x daily
	linden ⬤	3x daily			
	thyme ⬤	3x daily		thyme ⬤	As a douche 2 – 3x daily
Colic	chamomile ⬤	3x daily			
	chamomile ✕	3x daily			
	lemon balm ⬤	3x daily	Hay fever	elder ⬤	3x daily during hay-fever season
Coughs, chesty	elder ⬤	3x daily			
	garlic, fresh	3 – 5 cloves daily	Headache, tension	chamomile ⬤	3x daily
	ginger ⬤	3x daily		chamomile ✕	3x daily
	thyme ⬤	3x daily		linden ⬤	3x daily
	thyme ✕	3x daily	Hemorrhoids	calendula ⌀	2 – 3x daily
Coughs, irritable	plantain ⬤	3x daily		plantain ⌀	2 – 3x daily

There are many remedies that could be included in a natural medicine kit; those suggested here meet the criteria of being easily available and of having a wide range of uses. They are also especially safe for home use, but it is still important not to exceed the recommended doses outlined here. Infusions of chamomile, elder, linden flowers, and lemon balm are safe for all ages. However, with other remedies for internal use, children aged 3 to 10 should be given one third of the adult dose and children aged 11 to 16 should be given half the adult dose. Children under three are best not treated internally without professional advice. To use the remedy guide below, find the condition you want to treat in the ailment column, then look across to the next two columns for the choice of remedies and the dosages. Further details on how and when to use each remedy are on pp. 136–37.

Dosage symbols: ⬩ = one medicine spoonful   ᗺ = apply to the
       Ⲷ = ³/₄ of a cup   affected area

AILMENT	REMEDY	DOSAGE	AILMENT	REMEDY	DOSAGE
Indigestion	dandelion ⬩	10 – 15 daily	Rheumatic pain	arnica ⬡	6 or 12x 3x daily for 10 days
	dandelion ⬡⚗	Ⲷ 3x daily		feverfew ⬩	3 daily
	dandelion ⬟	⬩ 3x daily		feverfew capsules	As directed
	ginger ⬡	Ⲷ 3x daily	Shingles	lemon balm ⬟	Apply 2 – 3x daily
	lemon balm ⬡	Ⲷ 3x daily	Sinusitis	elder ⬡	Ⲷ 3x daily
	thyme ⬡	Ⲷ 3x daily		ginger ⬡	Ⲷ 3x daily
Insect bites and stings	apis ⬡	30x every 15 minutes for 6 doses	Skin infections	calendula ⬡ ⬟	ᗺ as a lotion 3x daily
Insomnia	chamomile ⬡	Ⲷ 3x daily		garlic, crushed	ᗺ 2 – 3x daily
	chamomile ⬟	⬩ 3x daily	Sprains	arnica ⬡	6 or 12x 3x daily for 10 doses
	lemon balm ⬡	Ⲷ 3x daily		arnica ▱	ᗺ 2 – 3x daily
	linden ⬡	Ⲷ 3x daily	Stomach infections	thyme ⬡	Ⲷ 3x daily
Lung infections	garlic, fresh	3 – 5 cloves daily	Sunburn	calendula ▱	ᗺ 2 – 3x daily
	thyme ⬡	Ⲷ 3x daily	Teething pain	chamomile ⬡	Ⲷ 3x daily
	thyme ⬟	⬩ 3x daily		chamomile ⬟	⬩ 3x daily
Menstrual cramps	feverfew ⬩	3 daily	Throat infections	elder ⬡	Ⲷ 3x daily
	feverfew capsules	As directed		garlic, fresh	3 – 5 cloves daily
Migraine	feverfew ⬩	3 daily during attacks; 1 daily to prevent attacks		plantain ⬡	Ⲷ 3x daily
				thyme ⬡	Ⲷ 3x daily
	feverfew capsules	As directed	Thrush (mouth and vaginal)	calendula ⬡	As a douche or mouthwash
Morning sickness	ginger ⬡	Ⲷ 3x daily		chamomile ⬡	
Motion sickness	ginger ⬡	Ⲷ 3x daily		thyme ⬡	2 – 3x daily
Muscle strain	arnica ⬡	6 or 12x 3x daily for 10 doses	Varicose ulcers	calendula ⬡	ᗺ as a lotion 2 – 3x daily
	arnica ▱	ᗺ 2 – 3x daily		garlic, crushed	ᗺ 2 – 3x daily
Nausea	chamomile ⬡	Ⲷ 3x daily		ginger ⬡	ᗺ as a lotion 2 – 3x daily
	chamomile ⬟	⬩ 3x daily		plantain ⬕	ᗺ 2 – 3x daily
	ginger ⬡	Ⲷ 3x daily	Warts	dandelion sap	ᗺ 2 – 3x daily
Nervous tension/ stress	chamomile ⬡	Ⲷ 3x daily		garlic juice	ᗺ 2 – 3x daily
	chamomile ⬟	⬩ 3x daily	Worms	garlic, fresh	3 – 5 cloves daily
	lemon balm ⬡	Ⲷ 3x daily		thyme ⬡	Ⲷ 3x daily
	linden ⬡	Ⲷ 3x daily			
Restlessness in children	chamomile ⬡	Ⲷ 3x daily			
	chamomile ⬟	⬩ 3x daily			
	linden ⬡	Ⲷ 3x daily			

APIS (*Apis mellifera*)
Insect stings and bites are classic examples of ailments that call for simple and immediate first aid. Homeopathic remedies for stings are popular. *Apis* is a homeopathic remedy made from honeybees and can be used for stings, bites, and other painful inflammatory conditions and swellings.

How to use
Tablets in different strengths can be purchased from a pharmacy or homeopathic shop.

ARNICA (*Arnica montana*)
Arnica is very poisonous if taken internally except in homeopathic doses. Arnica tablets, and cream (homeopathic or herbal), are suitable for painful bruises with swelling, and for relieving the pain of strained muscles, sprains, and rheumatism. The cream should not be applied to broken skin.

How to use
Both cream and different strength tablets can be purchased from a pharmacy or homeopathic shop.

CALENDULA/MARIGOLD (*Calendula officinalis*)
Calendula is one of the most useful wound herbs. It is excellent for cuts and abrasions and other surface wounds such as leg ulcers. It has a strong antimicrobial effect against bacteria, viruses, fungi, and many protozoa, and is a valuable treatment for athlete's foot, boils, and eye and skin infections. It is useful as a mouthwash or douche for oral or vaginal thrush respectively, and as an eyewash for eye infections. A tincture of calendula is particularly useful as a lotion for acne. In a cream, it is effective on minor burns, sunburn, eczema, and hemorrhoids.

How to use
Standard infusions, tinctures, poultices, and creams can be made from fresh or dried flower heads.

CHAMOMILE (*Matricaria recutita* or *Chamamaelum nobilis*)
A relaxing herb, it is particularly useful for anxiety and tension. It relieves tension headaches and nausea, colic, and flatulence due to stress. It is safe for young children, calming irritability, promoting sleep, and easing teething pains. It is anti-inflammatory and antiseptic and thus helpful for washing wounds, but is especially useful in the treatment of itching and weeping eczema. As a douche, it helps relieve vaginal thrush.

How to use
A standard infusion or tincture of flower heads is used internally, but only infusions should be used externally. Tea bags are widely available and make convenient poultices for eczema or wounds.

DANDELION (*Taraxacum officinalis*)
The leaves of this common weed are one of the most effective and useful diuretics known, helping with edema and water retention, especially that of premenstrual swelling of the breasts and feelings of pelvic bloating. The leaves and roots are bitters, which stimulate digestive function and help those who suffer from indigestion.

The root is a useful liver "tonic" and helps to increase the flow of bile, which is necessary for efficient digestion, especially of fatty diets. Herbalists use dandelion root to help the liver recover from diseases like jaundice, hepatitis, and cirrhosis. Dandelion sap, especially from the root, can help to remove warts.

How to use
The leaves can be eaten fresh from the garden, or dried and made into a standard infusion or tincture. The root should be harvested in the autumn, chopped finely, and taken as a standard decoction, or chopped and roasted to be used like coffee beans to make a useful caffeine-free alternative to coffee.

ELDER (*Sambucus nigra*)
This plant is almost a first-aid kit on its own. It dries up the running nose and streaming eyes of hay fever and, if taken before the pollen season begins, can reduce the severity of symptoms from the start. It also reduces catarrh and controls fever associated with the common cold, sinusitis, flu, and bronchitis. Externally, it eases fungal eye infections and soothes minor burns.

How to use
Fresh elder flowers are best but are only available for two or three weeks a year. They can be frozen or gently dried in an airing cupboard and made into a standard infusion.

FEVERFEW (*Tanacetum parthenium*)
Sufferers of migraines are used to being left to their own devices. Feverfew offers a proven remedy that can reduce the intensity of a migraine attack. It has also been found to be a useful preventive if taken before the telltale signs of blurred vision and nausea appear. In addition, feverfew helps relieve rheumatic and menstrual cramps.

How to use
Fresh or frozen leaves are best but dried herb in capsules is available from good herbal suppliers. The plant is attractive and is easily grown in a garden or indoors in a pot, so a steady supply throughout the year is possible. Some people may experience small mouth ulcers from chewing feverfew leaves. To avoid this, simply place a leaf in a small sandwich and chew it minimally before swallowing.

GARLIC (*Allium sativum*)
An excellent antimicrobial remedy for internal use, garlic kills organisms responsible for food poisoning, and it kills many common intestinal worms. In addition, the volatile oils it contains pass from the blood to the lungs, where they help disinfect the respiratory tract in bacterial throat and lung infections. Garlic is also an expectorant, helping to clear the chest in colds and bronchitis. Applied to boils, varicose ulcers, and skin infections, crushed garlic encourages healing and speeds the demise of any infection. Garlic juice from fresh cloves helps to remove viral warts.

How to use
Garlic is best fresh for both internal and external use. The characteristic breath odor comes from the active ingredients and is necessary for the best results. Commercial preparations such as oil-filled pearls or pills are available but are less effective than the fresh cloves. For

internal use, cloves can be eaten whole, crushed in honey, used in salad dressings, or made into a sandwich with parsley.

———— • ————

GINGER (*Zingiber officinalis*)
Ginger has a proven record of relieving motion sickness and morning sickness in pregnancy. It also stimulates the circulation of the feet and hands, which is helpful in conditions such as chilblains, varicose ulcers, and cold hands and feet in winter. This same action causes a healthy sweat in mild feverish conditions such as the common cold, and it produces watery mucus, which helps unblock stuffed-up noses in sinusitis and colds. Small amounts of ginger in food help to stimulate digestive juices, so helping to relieve indigestion and flatulence.

How to use
Fresh ginger root is best and is taken as a standard infusion. If fresh root is not available, use ground ginger, adding 1 1/2 teaspoons to 2 cups of water.

———— • ————

LEMON BALM (*Melissa officinalis*)
An excellent relaxing herb that promotes gentle sleep without addiction, lemon balm is suitable for calming restless children before bedtime. In adults, it helps relax a digestive system disturbed by nervous tension, and reduces colic and flatulence. Treat cold sores with a tincture of lemon balm.

How to use
Standard infusions or tinctures of fresh whole herb are best. Either use the herb fresh from the garden or harvest it just before flowering and freeze immediately Dried herb is available but is not as potent.

———— • ————

LINDEN (*Tilia* x *europea*)
Irritable children are readily and safely calmed by an infusion of linden flowers. It is also a notable relaxant for the stresses and anxieties of daily life and can be drunk at any time of the day without causing drowsiness or addiction. It helps relieve insomnia and tension headaches, and hastens recovery from flu and colds. Linden also has a lowering effect on the blood pressure, which can help anyone with a blood pressure at the higher end of the normal range. People prescribed medication by a doctor for their blood pressure should also benefit from linden, but they should not alter the dosage of prescribed drugs without professional advice.

How to use
A standard infusion should be prepared from dried linden flowers collected during the previous spring. Tea bags are available from good supermarkets and other suppliers of herbal infusions.

———— • ————

PLANTAIN (*Plantago major*)
The high mucilage content of plantain makes it an ideal soothing remedy. It eases sore throats and laryngitis, hoarseness from over-using the voice, and irritable coughs. Plantain poultices help heal wounds, especially varicose ulcers and other slow healing wounds. It soothes the intestines in gastritis (stomach inflammation), eases irritated urinary tubes in conditions like cystitis, and alleviates hemorrhoids.

How to use
Standard infusions and creams can be prepared from fresh or dried leaves. A poultice should be made from crushed leaves.

———— • ————

THYME (*Thymus* species)
Thyme from the garden or the spice rack has long been a useful respiratory and stomach remedy. Its volatile oil contains a strong antimicrobial, thymol, which helps in lung, throat, and stomach infections. It can be used to relieve the common cold and is an efficient expectorant, helping to clear catarrh from the lungs. This is aided by its ability to help relax spasms that narrow the small airways in the lungs, which eases breathing. Thyme also helps alleviate food poisoning and intestinal worms.

In addition, the volatile oil in thyme passes into the kidneys, where it helps to disinfect the urine and bladder in conditions like cystitis. The herb is also effective against fungal infections and can be used as a mouthwash against oral thrush, as a douche for vaginal thrush, and as a lotion for infections of the head, and of the feet, for example, athlete's foot.

How to use
A standard infusion or tincture can be prepared using fresh or dried whole herb. If you use an herb from your household spice rack, make sure that it was harvested in the previous year and that you do not keep it for more than a year.

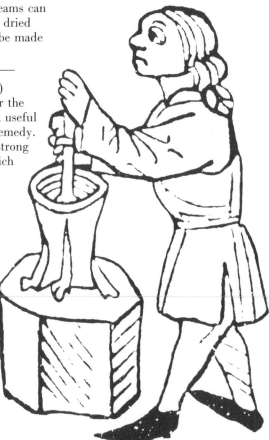

A 15th-century herbalist preparing a remedy.

Glossary

Alchemy. A medieval form of chemistry best known for attempting to transform common metals into gold.

Alkaloids. A group of medicinally useful plant compounds containing nitrogen molecules in ring structures.

Alterative. Stimulates the body's nutrition and elimination processes to greater efficiency.

Amino acids. Nitrogen-containing organic acids that form the basic building blocks of protein molecules.

Amoeba. A single-cell micro-organism that causes diseases such as dysentery.

Analgesic. Relieves pain.

Antacid. Neutralizes any excess stomach acid.

Anthelmintic. Kills and helps expel intestinal worms.

Anthraquinones. Important plant constituents which are useful laxatives and cathartics.

Anti-allergic. Prevents allergic reactions or reduces the symptoms.

Antibacterial. Destroys bacteria or inhibits their growth.

Anti-emetic. Suppresses nausea and vomiting.

Antifungal. Destroys fungi.

Anti-inflammatory. Reduces or prevents inflammation.

Antilithic. Prevents the formation of or aids the breakdown of kidney stones.

Antimicrobial. Destroys micro-organisms.

Anti-oxidant. Slows or stops the oxidation of substances.

Antiprozoal. Destroys protozoa.

Antipyretic. Helps reduce fever.

Antispasmodic. Reduces muscle tension and spasms.

Antitussive. Inhibits the cough reflex, helping to stop coughing.

Antiviral. Inhibits viral infection or the spread of a virus once in the body.

Aperient. Very mildly laxative.

Aromatic. A compound with a distinct smell or taste.

Astringent. Binds the proteins of mucous membranes and other body surfaces, producing a protective coating.

Auto-immune disease. A condition caused by the immune system attacking the body's own tissues and cells.

Bacteriocidal. Kills bacteria.

Bitter. A substance that stimulates the bitter taste buds on the tongue, resulting in the increased secretion of digestive juices and a heightened appetite.

Bulk laxative. A laxative that increases the rate of movement and volume of feces through the bowel by helping to produce large, soft stools.

Calyx. The sterile parts of a flower that surround the petals.

Carminitive. Relieves digestive colic and flatulence.

Carotenoids. Yellow or orange plant pigments which may be converted into vitamin A in the body.

Cathartic. Totally purges the bowels.

Caustic. Corrosive to body tissue.

Cholagogue. Increases the flow of bile from the liver.

Choleretic. Increases the production of bile in the liver.

Cholinergic. The part of the nervous system controlled by the chemical transmitter acetylcholine.

Circulatory stimulant. Increases blood flow by any of several influences on the heart or blood vessels.

Cold conditions. Disharmonies in Chinese medicine associated with an excess of Yin.

Colic. Acute spasmodic pain in the intestines or organs like the gallbladder.

Compound leaves. Leaves made up of several distinct and symmetrical parts joined to the stem via a common stalk.

Coumarins. Chemicals in grasses and legumes that provide anti-clotting drugs.

Counterirritant. Causes local irritation of the skin to give temporary relief of deeper inflammation and pain.

Demulcent. Softens and soothes body surfaces such as the digestive tract.

Detoxicant. Neutralizes toxins.

Diaphoretic. Induces sweating.

Diuretic. Increases urine production.

Emetic. Induces vomiting.

Emmenagogue. Stimulates menstrual flow.

Emollient. Softens and soothes skin.

Enzymes. Proteins that act as catalysts in specific biological reactions.

Essential oil. A volatile oil made up of many ingredients, that has been distilled from plant extracts.

Estrogen. A multifunctional group of hormones produced in the ovaries.

Expectorant. Encourages the softening and removal of phlegm and other material from the respiratory tract.

Fatty acids. The building blocks of the fats and oils in plants and animals.

Febrifuge. Reduces or prevents fever.

Fertile stem. A specialized reproductive stem on plants that also produces separate vegetative stems which provide food energy for the plant.

Flavonoids. A large group of plant constituents that contribute to plant dyes and have many healing actions.

Floret. Single flower units in compound floral structures, such as grass spikes or daisylike flower heads.

Follicle-stimulating hormone. A hormone released from the human pituitary gland which initiates growth of eggs in females and sperm in males.

Galls. Protective swellings that grow on leaves and stems of plants following irritation by burrowing insect larvae.

Glaucoma. A serious disease of the human eye caused by increased fluid pressure within the eye.

Glycosides. Medicinally useful plant substances containing sugar molecules which help keep them soluble.

Gonadotrophic hormones. Human hormones that stimulate both male and female gonads (sex glands).

Hot conditions. Disharmonies in Chinese medicine associated with an excess of Yang.

Hypotensive. Lowers blood pressure.

Immunostimulant. Stimulates and enhances the body's immune defenses.

Laxative. Increases the movement of feces through the bowel.

Liniment. A medication, usually containing rubefacient or antispasmodic remedies, that is rubbed on the skin to relieve muscular or joint pain.

Lipids. Fatlike substances, including fats, waxes, and phospholipids.

Luteinizing hormone. A hormone released from the human pituitary gland which initiates egg release and stimulates production of progesterone in ovaries and testosterone in testes.

Mucilages. Complex plant substances, made of polysaccharides, that are soft and slippery, and protect mucous membranes and inflamed tissues.

Mydriatic. Stimulates abnormal dilation of the pupil of the eye.

Nervine. Restores the nervous system and may also relax, sedate, or stimulate.

Neuralgia. Pain along a nerve.

Nutritive. Provides nutrients.

Over-the-counter. Pharmaceutical drugs available without a prescription.

Peripheral circulation. Blood supply to the outer regions of the body, such as the arms, legs, muscles, and skin.

Physiomedicalism. A system of herbalism developed in the 1800s in the United States by Samuel Thompson.

Polysaccharides. A large group of plant substances, such as starch, made up of chains of simple sugars.

Progesterone. A female hormone produced in the ovaries after egg release.

Prostaglandins. A group of hormonelike substances in the body that act as chemical messengers.

Proteolytic. Dissolves protein in dead skin, warts, corns, etc.

Protozoa. A class of single-celled organisms such as the malaria parasite.

Psoriasis. A chronic skin condition characterized by thick, silvery scales.

Purgative. Evacuates the bowel by producing liquid feces.

Rhizome. A swollen root.

Rubefacient. Stimulates blood flow to the skin, causing localized reddening.

Saponins. Complex organic compounds that produce a lather in water, but are more interesting for their similarity to steroids and hormones.

Sciatica. Pain in the parts of the leg and buttock served by the sciatic nerve.

Scurvy. Vitamin C deficiency disease.

Sedative. Reduces functional activity of organs and muscles, and calms over-excitement of the nervous system.

Stigma. The part of a flower that pollen contacts and enters when fertilizing the ova, or embryonic seeds.

Style. The part of a flower that protrudes from the ovary to receive pollen grains on its terminal stigma.

Styptic. Stops bleeding from wounds.

Tannins. Phenolic-rich constituents, found in barks, leaves, and galls, that are thought to protect plants from insects.

Thallus. The body of primitive plants such as lichens.

Thrombosis. A serious condition in which blood clots form within blood vessels and restrict flow.

Tisane. A weak tea or infusion made with boiling water.

Tonic. Restores tone to a system by nourishing, restoring, and supporting.

Trophorestorative. Supports the nutrition and tone of the nervous system to affect body function as a whole.

Tuber. A swollen underground plant stem, specialized for storage.

Urinary antiseptic. Disinfects the urinary tract.

Uterine tonic. Increases the tone of womb muscles and tissues.

Vasodilator. Increases the diameter of blood vessels.

Vegetative stem. See *fertile stem*.

Vulnerary. Promotes wound healing.

Bibliography

Bensky and Gamble: *Chinese Herbal Materia Medica*, Eastland Press, Seattle, WA 1986.
British Herbal Medicine Association: *British Herbal Pharmacopoeia*, Bournemouth, UK, 1983.
Castro, M.: *The Complete Homeopathy Handbook*, Macmillan, London, 1990.
Chishti, H.: *The Traditional Healer*, Inner Traditions International, Rochester, VT, 1988.
Grieve, M.: *A Modern Herbal*, Dover Publications, New York, 1978.
Heyn, B.: *Ayurvedic Medicine*, Thorsons, London, 1987.
Hunan Province, China Health Committee: *A Barefoot Doctor's Manual*, 1990.
Kaptchuk, T. and Croucher, M.: *The Healing Arts*, Summit Books, New York, 1987.
Lasak, E. V. and McCarthy, T.: *Australian Medicinal Plants*, Methuen, North Ryde, Australia, 1983.
Lockie, Dr. A.: *The Family Guide to Homeopathy*, Elm Tree Books, London, 1989.
Mabey, R. et al: *The New Age Herbalist*, Collier Books, New York, 1988.
McNeill, W. H.: *Plagues and Peoples*, Doubleday, New York, 1987.
Priest, A. W. and Priest, L. R.: *Herbal Medication: A Clinical and Dispensary Handbook*, Fowler, London, 1982.
Read, B. E.: *Chinese Materia Medica*, Oriental Book Store, Pasadena, CA, 1982.
Royal Pharmaceutical Society: *Martindale The Extra Pharmacopoeia*, 29th edition, London, 1989.
Stockwell, C.: *Nature's Pharmacy*, Random Century, North Pomfret, VT, 1988.
Trease, G. E. and Evans, W. C.: *Pharmacognosy*, 12th edition, Balliére Tindall, Philadelphia, PA, 1983.
Vohora, Dr. S. B.: *Animal Origin Drugs Used in Unani Medicine*, Advent NY, 1980.
Weiss, R. F.: *Herbal Medicine*, Medicina Bio, Portland, OR, 1988.
Wren, R. C.: *Potter's New Cyclopaedia of Botanical Drugs and Preparations*, Daniel, Saffron Walden, UK, 1988.

Index

Page numbers in **bold** refer to entries in the Reference Guide, which includes a history, the parts used, the active ingredients, the actions, the medicinal uses, and the preparations for each entry. Page numbers in *italics* refer to entries in the photographic Nature's Medicine Chest.

Acknowledgments

Authors' acknowledgments. Our most important helper has been Helen Barnett, our editor, who has contributed a rare knowledge of different forms of medicine, as well as skilled and sympathetic support. We also thank Dr. R. M. Ballentine, M.D., Helen Busby MNIMH, Kerri Caldock, Christopher Hedley MNIMH, Jeffrey McNeely of the World Conservation Union, Michael McIntyre MNIMH, Dr. Len Mervyn, Simon Mills MNIMH, Professor E. J. Shellard, and Hein Zeylstra FNIMH. The Wellcome Institute for the History of Medicine in London has been very useful.

Dorling Kindersley would like to thank Steve Painter for helping with design; Sarah Ashun for assisting at photography; Candace Burch for help with proofreading; Sue Bosanko for the index; Victoria Wood for tracking down props; Kew Gardens; Merck Limited; Natural History Museum; Novo Nordisk Pharmaceuticals Limited; William Ransom & Son.
  The following companies provided plants, animals, and/or minerals for photography: Culpeper Limited, Hadstock Road, Linton, Cambridge CB1 6NJ; East West Herb Shop, 2 Neal's Yard, London WC2H 9DP; Gregory Bottley & Lloyd, 8-12 Rickett Street, London SW6 1RU; Hambleden Herbs, Hambleden, Henley-on Thames, Oxfordshire RG9 6SX; Hollington Nurseries, Woolton Hill, Newbury, Berkshire, RG15 9XT; Poyntzfield Herb Nursery, Black Isle, By Dingwall, Ross & Cromarty, Scotland IV7 8LX; Suffok Herbs, Sawyers Farm, Little Cornard, Sudbury, Suffolk IP33 1NX.

Key to illustration positions: t = top; b= bottom; l = left; r = right

ILLUSTRATORS
David Ashby: pp. 34, 40
Colette Cheng: p. 11r
Sarah Ponder: pp. 59, 94, 107, 110, 112, 116, 119, 124, 125

PICTURE CREDITS
All photography by Steve Gorton except for:
Bodleian Library, Oxford (MS. Ashmole 1462): pp. 14t, 16b; The Bridgeman Art Library, London: pp. 16t, 20tl; British Library (010C): pp. 12b, 26tl; Dorling Kindersley: p. 19; The Mansell Collection: p. 10b; Mary Evans Picture Library: pp. 13t, 14b, 17, 18b, 19t, 24t; National Maritime Museum, London: p. 15b; © Photo Michael Holford: pp. 10t, 13b; Photographer/Aspect Picture Library: p. 22tl; Photographer/Science Photo Library: p. 28tl; Werner Forman Archive/Plains Indian Museum, Wyoming: p. 18t.